Understanding Autoimmune Disease And Stress-Related Illness

(a guide for laypersons and healthcare professionals)

Uncovering the Mystery

Copyright © 2009 by Brucene Wilson

Lulu Publishing Inc.
Raleigh, NC 27612

All rights reserved. No part of this book may be reproduced in any form or by any electronic or mechanical means, including information storage and retrieval systems, without permission in writing from the publisher, except by a reviewer who may quote brief passages in a review.

First Edition

This book is not meant to diagnose or treat in anyway. Consult your personal physician before beginning any new medicine, diet or exercise.

Library of Congress Cataloging-in-Publication Data
Wilson, Brucene Renae
      Understanding Autoimmune Disease and Stress-Related Illness/ Brucene Wilson.—1st ed.

      p. cm.

ISBN 978-0-557-11026-1

Acknowledgements

*This book is dedicated to
Mary Margaret Hackney and
Earl James Hackney for their dedication,
sacrifice and belief in me;
to my parents, Earlene and Bruce Wilson,
for all their help;
to Roy Thompson for his wonderful editing.
And to all those who suffer from these ailments and
rise above their circumstances.*

Content

Chapter 1: The Plague of the Modern World 12
The Most Commonly Diagnosed Autoimmune Diseases and Stress-Related Illnesses
Rheumatoid Arthritis, Multiple Sclerosis, Lupus, Fibromyalgia and Chronic Fatigue Syndrome

Chapter 2: The Stress Response 30
Hormones, The Nervous System, and You

Chapter 3: Vaccines, Germs, and Trauma 44

Chapter 4: Human Behavior and Disease 58

Chapter 5: Childhood Abuse, Neglect, and Stress-Related Illness 66

Part II: Autoimmune Disease and Stress-Related Survival

Chapter 6: Diagnosis and Treatments for Healthcare Professionals 76

Chapter 7: Feeling Better: A Maintenance Plan 101

Chapter 8: Stop the Madness: Exercise and Diet 112

Chapter 9: Preferred Psychotherapies for Individuals and Families with Autoimmune Disease and Stress-Related Illness 121

Chapter 10: Additional Resources 138

Introduction

The National Institutes of Health (NIH) estimates up to 23.5 million Americans have an autoimmune disease. In comparison, cancer affects up to nine million and heart disease up to 22 million.

The NIH estimates annual direct health-care costs for autoimmune disease to be in the range of $100 billion (source: NIH presentation by Dr. Fauci, NIAID). In comparison, cancer costs are $57 billion, and heart and stroke costs are $200 billion.

The NIH research funding for autoimmune disease in 2003 came to $591 million. In comparison, cancer funding came to $6.1 billion and heart and stroke to $2.4 billion.

The NIH Autoimmune Diseases Research Plan states: "Research discoveries of the last decade have made autoimmune research one of the most promising areas of new discovery."

Autoimmune disease is described differently by a variety of health professionals. It is a misinformed, malfunctioning immune system that has misinterpreted an incoming antigen. Autoimmune disease can be described as the immune system losing its ability to distinguish friend (self) from foe (foreign antigens). When this happens, the artillery of the immune system may turn against itself, like friendly fire during a war. That is, the body produces antibodies (autoantibodies) and sensitized cytotoxic T-cells that destroy its own tissues. This puzzling phenomenon is called autoimmune disease.

The most commonly reported autoimmune diseases are: Grave's disease, insulin-dependent diabetes mellitus, pernicious anemia, rheumatoid arthritis, thyroiditis, vitiligo, glomerulonehphritis, multiple sclerosis, and lupus. Some forms of stress-related illness that may include everything from chronic fatigue and fibromyalgia to high blood pressure and irritable bowel syndrome will affect more people than autoimmune disease.

The statistics revealed by the American Autoimmune Related Diseases Association (*AARDA*) are why it is important to investigate some of the possible relationships and triggers that may preclude these illnesses, so early prevention or intervention may be promptly initiated. Autoimmune diseases and stress-related illnesses are strongly associated with vaccines, trauma, germs, childhood abuse, neglect, and mental disorders. Moreover, psychotherapy promises to provide powerful means of coping with and perhaps relieving symptoms of some of these diseases.

This comprehensive analysis directed toward healthcare professionals and those affected by these illnesses, questions the origins, triggers and possible causes of autoimmune diseases and stress-related illnesses. Through extensive research, it is clear that autoimmune diseases and stress-related illnesses are far from being understood and even further from being cured. By definition of the American Arthritis Foundation and the National Institutes of Health, literally hundreds of illnesses can be categorized as autoimmune diseases and at least double that for stress-related illnesses. So in the interest of time and predominance, only the most commonly diagnosed autoimmune diseases are discussed, which include rheumatoid arthritis (RA), multiple sclerosis (MS), and lupus. The stress-related illnesses include: fibromyalgia and chronic fatigue syndrome (CFS).

    This book investigates the origins of these illnesses, and also provides an analysis as to what autoimmune diseases, and stress-related illnesses are and what may contribute to them. For example, *The Stress Response* chapter, focuses the bodies' reactions to everyday life and illness and how that may contribute or cause these diseases. Following *The Stress Response* chapter, is *Vaccines, Germs and Trauma*, which investigates the possible causes or contributors to these illnesses involving vaccines, viral and bacterial infections and traumas such as car accidents.

    Furthermore, the chapter on *Human Behavior and Disease*, explores how to possibly avoid getting many of the illnesses covered in the *Vaccines, Germs, and Trauma* chapter. In addition, the chapter on *Childhood Abuse and Neglect,* deals with childhood abuse and its association with developing stress-related illness in adulthood as another possible trigger, which could further lead to a stress-response cycle. Additionally, the subsequent chapter on *Autoimmune Disease, Stress-Related*

Illness, and Mental Disorders, investigates how mental disorders play a role in these illnesses.

And one of the most defining chapters in this book, *Psychotherapies Commonly Used for Autoimmune Disease and Stress-Related Illness*, helps the individuals facing chronic illness in their life or the life of a loved one better cope with their diagnosis.

This information on autoimmune disease and stress-related illness is very timely. It has come in an age where the threat of more and more required vaccinations is on the horizon due to increased disease factors and bio-terrorism. At almost no other time in our history other than around the time of World War II, has the threat of homeland security been more eminent.

Lastly, this book provides greater insights into autoimmunity and the vaccines, germs, trauma, childhood abuse, neglect and mental disorders that could be deleterious if there is a genetic predisposition for developing autoimmune disease and stress-related illness. This book will provide insights into understanding how to control the patient's illness through psychotherapy, and understanding the possible origins, triggers and causes of their illness.

Chapter 1

The Plague of the Modern World: The Most Commonly Diagnosed Autoimmune Diseases and Stress-Related Illnesses:

Rheumatoid Arthritis, Lupus, Multiple Sclerosis, Fibromyalgia and Chronic Fatigue Syndrome

My exploration of these illnesses starts at the very beginning with a young man named Allen. I first met Allen when he was a student at the college where I taught. He worked in the college gym as a trainer who helped me when I was in need of weight training. He appeared strong and healthy. We would talk at length about how he loved to run marathons and bike. One day I entered the gym to lift weights and he wasn't there. I later caught up with him and he explained to me that he had been diagnosed with multiple sclerosis (MS). He was devastated by his diagnosis, which was still in its infancy. This enthusiastic athlete now appeared terrified and dismal. His denial was evident when he spoke of continuing his workout routine, which was a rigorous routine only fit for a marathoner.

Allen's story begins in high school, where he was described as wild and reckless. When he was 17, and in prime physical condition, he was afflicted by a severe bout of mononucleosis and as a result, he was bedridden for several

weeks. As a result of his illness, he was unable to enter the Marine Corp as he had planned. He had lost almost 30 pounds and was hospitalized from the severe
symptoms he experienced, which included: sore throat, fever, and swollen glands. The mono turned quickly into strep throat and acute tonsillitis. After his recovery from this illness, he started experiencing severe fatigue and depression.

But Allen recovered and found the strength to graduate high school and enter college even after his Marine Corp disappointment. However, after he turned 20, he started having numbness in his left cheek sporadically. The symptoms progressed after his 21st birthday from a numb cheek to numbness in his entire right hand. Following these symptoms, Allen began to have the classical problems with vision that most MS patients experience. He described one day as everything being blurred and difficult to see.

When the symptoms worsened he sought the advice of a neurologist, who after several MRI's and multiple other tests, diagnosed him with MS. Also revealed that prior to his illness with mono, he also had an appendectomy and was involved in several car accidents, which resulted in concussions and neck contusions.

His history with mono and the multiple car accidents certainly piqued my interest as a possible trigger if not cause of his MS. It was also striking to me that he has no family history of

Understanding Autoimmune Disease and Stress-Related Illness

MS or any other autoimmune disease. Also interesting is the fact that men suffer from autoimmune disease one-third less as much as women. All of these factors led me to begin thinking about the possible connections that illness and trauma could play as possible factors in
the triggering or causation of autoimmune disease and stress-related illness.

It is also worth noting that while interviewing Allen for this book, I was in my own recovery from doctors diagnosing me with everything from rheumatoid arthritis to fibromyalgia. I had a history of prior illness and auto accidents as well as a hysterectomy that preceded my "autoimmune" symptoms. My specific case will be discussed more in following chapters.

After deciding to write about these topics, I met a woman who had been diagnosed with fibromyalgia. My journey with Beth began like many of the other cases I investigated. She explained about her medical history and psychological history, as both were equally as important for the sake of my research.

Beth revealed to me many precipitating events that were similar to my stories prior to her diagnosis with fibro. She also experienced long bouts of depression following illness and several car accidents. She, like Allen had also experienced mono and continued to test with very high Epstein-Barr virus (EBV) antibody titers indicating her immune system may be misfiring. Another connection that my case had with hers, in addition to a couple of car accidents, several surgeries and illness, she had received Hepatitis A and B vaccines.

She began to experience symptoms of fibromyalgia soon after her last Hepatitis B inoculation. She described her symptoms after the vaccine as "flu" like. Her body ached so severely that on
most days she was unable to get out of bed. Shortly after all of the "flu" like symptoms developed, she experienced severe and debilitating fatigue that the doctors later diagnosed as chronic fatigue syndrome. She was later diagnosed as having bi-polar disorder (formerly known as manic depression).

Others had similar stories, such as Norma. She facilitated a local fibromyalgia support group in her local community. Norma, diagnosed with Rheumatoid Arthritis (RA) and fibromyalgia like many of the others and myself, had an extensive history of car accidents, illness and surgeries. Like Beth, she was diagnosed first with many bouts of severe depression and then later as having bi-polar disorder.

One common thread that continued to reemerge in all of these interviews was the ongoing story of Hepatitis B vaccinations and a prior trauma that precipitated the onset of autoimmune symptoms. Sara was diagnosed with lupus after her second child had been born. She too had received a Hepatitis B vaccine in her twenties before having her first child. Sara started feeling some of the symptoms then, but wasn't conclusively diagnosed until she was bedridden with swollen joints and pleurisy in her lungs at the age of 30, two weeks after her second child was born. Sara had multiple reproductive problems that included endometriosis, which required seven laproscopic surgeries to remove the lesions, and in between the surgeries, she was put on Lupron injections. Like me, she went through Lupron injections to control her reproductive symptoms, which puts most women into an immediate menopause while on the injections. However, because she wanted children, she continued on the Lupron injections instead of having a hysterectomy.

      While working with the developmentally disabled in her twenties, a client assaulted Sara during a psychotic break and threw her into a wall damaging her shoulder, knocking her unconscious and resulting in a severe concussion. As a result of this incident, she needed shoulder surgery. In addition to having a child, an injury and a Hepatitis B vaccine as a result of working with the developmentally disabled, her medical merry-go-round was just beginning. In addition, almost everyone in her family had been diagnosed with an autoimmune disease.

      Other women interviewed were diagnosed with a range of autoimmune diseases and stress-related illnesses had at least half of these symptoms in common including: emotional or physical trauma, car accidents, illness, surgeries (mostly reproductive), and vaccines as well as a diagnosis of depression, anxiety, and/or bi-polar disorder.

Through these interviews and case histories, I concluded that all these factors play a pivotal role in the development of autoimmune disease and stress-related illness. So, before going any further into my investigations as to the triggers and possible causes of autoimmune disease and stress-related illness, I feel the most commonly diagnosed autoimmune and stress-related illnesses must be thoroughly defined, which include: multiple sclerosis (MS), rheumatoid arthritis (RA), lupus, fibromyalgia (FMS) and chronic fatigue syndrome (CFS).

What does autoimmune mean?

An estimated 5 percent of adults in North America are afflicted with autoimmune disease. To further define each of the above commonly diagnosed autoimmune diseases, let's first look at multiple sclerosis.

Multiple Sclerosis:

According to medical experts, multiple sclerosis is a disease characterized by visual disturbances (including blindness), problems controlling muscles (weakness, clumsiness), and urinary incontinence. In this disease, myelin sheaths in the central nervous system (CNS) are gradually destroyed, reduced to nonfunctional hardened sheaths called scleroses. The loss of myelin (due to immune attack on myelin basic protein) results in such substantial shunting and short-circuiting of the current that successive nodes are excited more and more slowly, and eventually impulse conduction ceases. However, the axons themselves are not damaged and growing numbers of sodium channels appear spontaneously in the demyelinated fibers. This may account for the remarkably variable cycles of exacerbation and remission that are typical of this disease. And unlike some other autoimmune diseases, MS has very specific cycles that include:

- Approximately 5 percent will see their symptoms rapidly worsen.
- About 15 percent of sufferers will have intermittent periods of symptoms that grow progressively worse.
- An estimated 20 percent have essentially no impact and few symptoms.
- Some 60 percent of MS sufferers will experience intermittent symptoms, interspersed with periods of normal health.
- And about 15 percent will need substantial care and may be confined to a wheelchair.

Symptoms may include:

- Numbness
- Tingling
- Other abnormal sensations
- Visual disturbances
- Difficulty in reaching orgasm, lack of sensation in the vagina, sexual impotence in men
- Dizziness or vertigo
- Weakness, clumsiness
- Difficulty in walking or maintaining balance
- Tremor
- Double vision
- Problems with bowel or bladder control, constipation
- Stiffness, unsteadiness, unusual tiredness

Rheumatoid Arthritis:

    According to the National Institute of Arthritis and Musculoskeletal and Skin Disease (NIAMS), rheumatoid arthritis is a chronic inflammatory disorder with an insidious onset. Though its onset is between the ages of 40 and 50, it may occur at any age much like MS and other autoimmune diseases. It affects three times as many women as men. While not as common as osteoarthritis, rheumatoid arthritis affects millions. It occurs in more than 1 percent of Americans. In the early stages of

RA, joint tenderness and stiffness are common. Many joints, particularly the small joints of the fingers, wrist, ankles, and feet, are afflicted at the same time and bilaterally. For example, if the right elbow is affected, most likely the left elbow is also affected. The course of RA is variable and marked by flare-ups (exacerbations) and remissions. Other illness can coincide with RA like osteoporosis, anemia, muscle atrophy, and cardiovascular problems. It has been theorized that streptococcus bacterium--the bacteria that can cause strep throat--may be suspect among many other viruses and bacteria that will be addressed in further chapters.

RA begins with inflammation of the synovial membrane of the affected joints, but ultimately all of the joint tissues may become involved. Without treatment, synovial fluid accumulates, causing joint swelling, and inflammatory cells to migrate into the joint cavity from the blood. In time, the joint is eroded and deformity may follow.

Symptoms of RA may include:

- Stiffness in the morning that lasts for more than one hour for at least six weeks
- Inflammation in three or more joints for at least six weeks
- Arthritis in the hand, wrist, or finger joints for at least six weeks
- Rheumatoid factor in the blood

- Characteristic changes on x-rays
- Joints tender to the touch
- Reduced range of motion
- Skin bumps called rheumatoid nodules, located near joints
- Swollen lymph nodes
- Low-grade fever
- Dry eyes
- Dry mouth
- Weakness
- Weight Loss
- Anemia
- Elevated Erythrocyte Sedimentation Rate (ESR)

Lupus:

According to the NIAMS, lupus is a chronic inflammatory disease that can affect many of the body's organs. Lupus produces inflammation of the skin, blood vessels, joints, and other tissues.

This disease was named lupus, which means "wolf," because many people who get it develop a butterfly-shaped rash over the cheeks and nose that gives them something of a wolf like appearance. At least 90 percent of those who contract lupus are

Understanding Autoimmune Disease and Stress-Related Illness

women, and women of Asian background appear to be at greater risk of developing lupus than other women. It usually develops between the ages of fifteen and thirty-five, although it may occur at any age.

According to the NIAMS, there are two types of lupus: systemic lupus erythematosus (SLE) and discoid lupus erythematosus (DLE). As the name implies, SLE is a systemic disease that affects many different parts of the body. The severity can range from mild to life threatening. The first symptoms of many cases of SLE resemble those of arthritis, with swelling and pain in the fingers and other joints. The disease may also appear suddenly, with acute fever. The characteristic red rash may appear across the cheeks; there may also be red, scaling lesions elsewhere on the body. Sores may form in the mouth. The lungs and kidneys are often involved. Approximately 50 percent of those with SLE develop nephritis, inflammation of the kidneys. In serious cases, the brain, lungs, spleen, and/or heart may be affected. SLE can cause anemia and inflammation of the surface membranes of the increased susceptibility to infection. If the central nervous system is involved, seizures, amnesia, psychosis, and deep depression may be present.

According to medical experts, the discoid type of lupus is a less serious disease that primarily affects the skin. And, the characteristic butterfly rash forms over the nose and cheeks. There may also be lesions elsewhere, commonly on the scalp and ears, and these lesions may recur or persist for years. The lesions are small, soft yellowish lumps. When they disappear, they often leave scars. If these scars form on the scalp, permanent bald patches may result. While DLE is not necessarily dangerous to overall health, it is a chronic and disfiguring skin disease. Some experts have related it to a reaction to infection with tubercle bacillus.

Both types of lupus follow a pattern of periodic flare-ups alternating with periods of remission. Exposure to the sun's ultraviolet rays can result in a flare-up of DLE and may even induce the first attack. Fatigue, pregnancy, childbirth, infection, stress, unidentified viral infections, and chemicals may also trigger a flare-up. Drug-induced cases usually clear up when the drug is discontinued, according to medical experts.

According to the American Rheumatism Association, four of the following eight symptoms must occur, either serially or at the same time, before a diagnosis can be made:

- Abnormal cells in the urine
- Arthritis
- Butterfly rash on the cheeks
- Sun sensitivity
- Mouth sores
- Seizures or psychosis

- Low white blood cell count, low platelet count, or hemolytic anemia
- The presence in the blood of a specific antibody that is found in 50 percent of people with lupus.

Fibromyalgia:

Fibromyalgia, which has not yet been identified as an autoimmune disorder, identified only by the American Autoimmune Related Diseases Association (AARDA) as autoimmune in nature, is a rheumatic disorder, possibly stress-related and characterized by chronic achy muscular pain that has no obvious physical cause. Most people feel the greatest affects of fibromyalgia in the lower back, neck, shoulders, the back of the head, upper chest, and/or the thighs, although any area or areas of the body may be involved.

Many people find it difficult to rise out of bed normally in the morning without a great deal of time and effort. The pain and stiffness of fibromyalgia can also be accompanied by headaches, strange sensations in the skin, insomnia, irritable bowel syndrome, and temporomandibular joint syndrome (TMJ).

According to medical experts, other symptoms often experienced by people with fibromyalgia include:
- Premenstrual syndrome (PMS)
- Painful periods

- Anxiety and palpitations
- Memory impairment
- Irritable bladder
- Skin sensitivities
- Dry eyes and mouth
- A need for frequent changes in eyeglass prescription
- Dizziness
- Impaired coordination

People who were once active begin to find simple activities such as climbing stairs or cleaning become difficult and painful. Depression is frequently part of the picture as well. However, often the most distinctive feature of fibromyalgia are the "tender points"—nine pairs of specific spots where the muscles are abnormally tender to the touch:

- Around the lower vertebra of the neck
- At the insertion of the second rib
- Around the upper part of the thigh bone
- In the middle of the knee joint
- In muscles connected to the base of the skull
- In muscles of the neck and upper back
- In muscles of the mid-back

- On the side of the elbow
- In the upper and outer muscles of the buttocks

There are 18 tender points specifically and if you have 11 out of 18, you may have a diagnosis of fibromyalgia, according to medical experts. Most people with fibromyalgia also have an associated sleep disorder known as alpha-EEG anomaly. In this disorder, the individual's deep sleep periods are interrupted by bouts of waking-type brain activity, resulting in poor sleep.

Furthermore, this disorder is much more common in females than in males, and most often begins in young adulthood. In most cases, symptoms come on gradually and slowly increase in intensity. In the majority of cases, symptoms are severe enough to interfere with normal daily activities; a significant number of people with fibromyalgia are disabled by the condition. The course of the disorder is unpredictable. Some cases clear up on their own, some become chronic, and some go through cycles of flare-ups alternating with periods of apparent remission.

Chronic Fatigue Syndrome:

Chronic Fatigue Syndrome (CFS)--identified by the AARDA as autoimmune in nature--like fibromyalgia has yet to be specifically identified as an autoimmune disease by the medical community—may be stress-related, and is a condition that has become wide spread in the United States. Symptoms associated with CFS are close to fibromyalgia and in some medical circles CFS is referred to as CFIDS, which stands for Chronic Fatigue Immune Dysfunction Syndrome.

Individuals with CFS may experience:
- Aching muscles and joints
- Anxiety
- Depression
- Difficulty concentrating
- Fever
- Headaches
- Intestinal problems
- Irritability
- Jaundice
- Loss of appetite
- Mood swings
- Muscle spasms
- Recurrent upper respiratory tract infections
- Sensitivity to light and heat
- Sleep disturbances
- Sore throat
- Swollen glands
- Temporary memory loss
- Extreme and often disabling fatigue

The symptoms of this syndrome resemble those of the flu and other viral infections, so it is often mistaken for other disorders. It is often misdiagnosed as hypochondria, psychosomatic illness, or depression, because routine medical tests may not detect these problems. The syndrome is three times more prevalent in women than in men, and primarily affects young adults between the ages of 20 and 40, according to medical experts.

The major criteria used to distinguish chronic fatigue syndrome are:

- Persistent fatigue that does not resolve with bed rest and that is severe enough to reduce average daily activity by at least 50 percent for at least six months.
- The presence of other chronic clinical conditions, including psychiatric disorders, can be ruled out.

The causes of chronic fatigue syndrome are not well understood. Some experts believe it is linked to infection with the Epstein-Barr virus (EBV), a member of the herpes virus family that is also the cause of mononucleosis. This belief is based in large part on the fact that many people with CFS have been found to have high levels of EBV antibodies in their blood, and that many people date the onset of symptoms to a prolonged bout with a viral infection. However, no connection between EBV and CFS has ever been conclusively proven. In addition many medical experts and scientists agree that most of the population has been exposed to EBV. Some healthy individuals have high EBV antibody titers and some CFS patients don't have high EBV titers, so it can't be conclusively linked as a possible trigger to CFS. It has also been postulated that several different types of herpes viruses could cause CFS, but again most of the population has been exposed and formed antibodies to various herpes viruses without CFS symptoms.

Lastly, according to medical experts, CFS is not life threatening, but may continue throughout life. Some people appear to recover spontaneously, but once this condition presents itself, it can recur at any time, usually following a bout with another illness or during times of stress.

Chapter 2

The Stress Response:

Hormones, The Nervous System, and You

A woman lifts a car off her child's crushed body, a man with MS runs across a burning bridge to save a loved one and the most vividly poignant story is a man during the 9/11 crisis in the World Trade Center ran up several flights of stairs to save fellow employees. You may have asked yourself, how one is able to keep going through insurmountable stress, and not stop to feel tired despite not having slept more than a few hours a night. The answer is the stress response.

Our bodies are incredibly adaptive to many different threats that could range from a bear in the woods to a germ in the air. It is our body's instinct to adapt to any environmental threat through our stress response. While our body doesn't know the difference between a perceived threat and a real threat, it mobilizes in order to meet the demands of any threat. We will examine how the body mobilizes itself through the nervous and endocrine systems.

To start, it is a complex interplay between the nervous system and endocrine system (hormones) that begs for further investigation. This interplay of hormones and the nervous system

The Stress Response

is what gives us that feeling of excitement or extra strength when something threatening could be approaching. The body begins to mobilize by producing hormones in a "fight-or-flight" situation. Hormones such as adrenaline and cortisol give us greater strength and acuity. It is all these different interactions between the nervous system and hormones that cause the heart to beat fast, palms to start sweating, and shortness of breath. Nausea and gastrointestinal symptoms such as diarrhea can be expected in times of extreme stress.

To explain the complicated interplay of these bodily functions, we must first look toward the hypothalamus, which regulates the master gland known as the pituitary gland. The pituitary gland is a pea-sized gland located in the area of the brain called the limbic system, which is also referred to as our emotional brain.

According to medical experts, the hypothalamus-pituitary-adrenal (HPA) axis is connected in many ways in the dispersal of different hormones in response to stress. This dispersal happens under varying degrees of stress, whether it's from the excitement of going out on that first date with someone new or because a burglar is threatening your life.

The HPA axis, in times of stress sends messages to different organs through the central nervous system and autonomic system, which mobilizes the peripheral nervous system's sympathetic system. When this occurs, our adrenal glands begin to release adrenaline and noradrenaline also known as norepinephrine and epinephrine, respectively. Adrenaline is what gives us the extra burst of energy that is needed in order to escape danger or perceived danger. The possibility of a mother lifting the car off her baby comes from the sudden rush of adrenaline that she would receive in that time of extreme panic. It is a basic survival mechanism in place to keep us alive and out of harm in order to continue the human race.

However, eventually our mind and body realizes we are no longer in any danger; this is when the parasympathetic part of the nervous system kicks into gear, calming the mind and body back to its original homeostasis. Adrenaline is a very fast-acting hormone that is useful during trying times and it is eliminated from the tissues of the body rapidly after its need has diminished.

As the HPA axis notifies the adrenal organs to release adrenaline, the hypothalamus and pituitary glands are also sending messages from the brain to glands to release glucocorticoids, which include many different types of stress hormones that are not easily diminished from the body after the stressful event has occurred.

The adrenal gland acts on the executive hypothalamus-pituitary (HP) orders from your stress response and we are off to the races. One of the main HP hormones released is corticotropin releasing factor (CRF), which then quickly triggers the pituitary to release the hormone ACTH also known as corticotropin. After this cycle ensues, the adrenal glands begin releasing glucocorticoid hormones like cortisol.

Cortisol is the enemy of all enemies hormonally. The release of cortisol from the adrenals begins a ripple effect in the body that taxes the immune system and many other organs, including our bones.

Cortisol has been linked to causing severe osteoporosis in adult women who have had no other risk factors. Often times, the cycle of stress and the release of the glucocorticoids in women in their twenties has been shown to cause significant bone loss preceding menopause.

Furthermore, glucocorticoids suppress the autonomic (vegetative), endocrine, immunologic and psychic responses to stressful stimuli. There are certainly physiological, and biochemical connections between osteoporosis and major depressive disorder (MDD). Both conditions are associated with a hyperactive HPA axis and as a result an increased CRH, and cortisol secretion occurs.

Recent research studies conducted by the division of endocrinology, diabetes and metabolic diseases at University Hospital in Croatia, demonstrated that earlier history of MDD was associated with marked osteoporosis. In MDD there are two well-documented biochemical abnormalities: hypercortisolism and its resistance to dexamethasone suppression. The study included 31 MDD patients (19 males and 12 females,), and 17 healthy male volunteers between the ages of 35 and 45. In each of the patients 24-hour cortisol, and a bone mineral density were measured. In addition, a group of young women with normal menstrual cycles, who were without signs of osteoporosis in the beginning, and who received anti-depressive therapy for many years were analyzed. Analysis showed that increased levels of cortisol and the occurrence of osteoporosis resulted.

In addition, in stress-related illnesses such as chronic fatigue syndrome and fibromyalgia, medical experts feel that the ongoing chronically elevated cortisol levels may lead to muscleskelatal pain and fatigue.

Furthermore, it is relevant to look at the implications of the HPA axis stress response on autoimmune disease and stress-related illness. It has long been theorized by medical doctors and researchers that stress in any form may play a pivotal role in triggering autoimmunity or at the very least exacerbating the symptoms of individuals who are already experiencing autoimmunity.

Stress plays a role in many disease states including autoimmune disease and stress-related illness.

Like the case studies of Norma and Beth, the precipitating events leading to an autoimmune diagnosis may include some form of mental illness. After being diagnosed with such illnesses, the stress cycle ensues and the mental health of the patient could be compromised even further.

The Stress Response

There is evidence to support these theories of stress and mental illness playing key roles in autoimmune disease and stress-related illness. A study from University Hospital in Regensburg, Germany, suggests a serious connection between the HPA axis and autoimmune illness. The study suggests a dysfunction of the HPA axis, which was found in animal models of chronic inflammatory diseases, and the defect was located in more central portions of the HPA axis. This defect of the neuroendocrine regulatory mechanisms was determined to contribute to a disease state. Since these first observations in animal models were made, evidence has accumulated that the possible defect in the HPA axis in humans is more distal to the hypothalamus or pituitary gland: In chronic inflammatory diseases, such as rheumatoid arthritis, an alteration of the HPA stress response results in inappropriately low cortisol secretion in relation to ACTH secretion. It has been shown that the serum levels of another adrenal hormone, dehydroepiandrosterone (DHEA), were significantly lower after ACTH stimulation in patients with rheumatoid arthritis. These studies clearly indicate that chronic inflammation alters, particularly, the adrenal response. However, at this point, the reason for the specific alteration of adrenal function in relation to pituitary function remains to be determined. Since one of the down-regulated adrenal hormones, DHEA can have an affect on immunity, low levels of this hormone may be deleterious in chronic inflammatory diseases. It has been demonstrated that DHEA is a potent inhibitor of immunity. DHEA affected B lymphocyte differentiation and tumor necrosis factors, which lead to disregulation of the immune system, which may be a significant risk factor in rheumatic diseases. And furthermore, the hormone DHEA also has played a key role in osteoporosis.

Due to the nature of most autoimmune diseases, the chronic use of steroids like Prednisone and different types of chemotherapy drugs further exacerbate adrenal burnout. This can cause severe symptoms when the patient takes a break from these medications, which forces them to get back on medication and so the cycle ensues.

In addition to all these factors, researchers have also recently identified the importance that a positive attitude can have on our immune system and stress-response. A study by Carnegie-Mellon University in Pittsburgh, concluded individuals who are tense and negative tend to get colds far more frequently and severely. Adults who scored the worst on calmness and positive mood were three times more likely to get colds and other illnesses. Those people who were considered extroverts were also much less likely to catch a cold than were the introverts. This correlates to friendship and social support as a powerful weapon against not only depression and loneliness, but also against illness. Scientists have found that daily moods and illness have a huge impact on our everyday health and stress levels. In a three-month study of daily moods and illness, adults had more antibodies to infection on days with positive events. The worse the day, the fewer antibodies, researchers found.

It would serve the patient's interest to attempt many additional, perhaps less harmful, alternative approaches to their symptoms in order to avoid a vicious cycle of illness.

The following is a stress and anxiety test to help you analyze whether stress is impeding your well-being:

In the past 12 months, which of the following major life events have taken place in your life.

1. Print out this form

2. Make a check mark next to each event that you have experienced this year.

3. When you're done, add up the points for each event.

4. Check your score at the bottom.

Understanding Autoimmune Disease and Stress-Related Illness

_____ **Death of Spouse 100**

_____ **Divorce 73**

_____ **Marital Separation 65**

_____ **Jail Term 63**

_____ **Death of close family member 63**

_____ **Personal injury or illness 53**

_____ **Marriage 50**

_____ **Fired from work 47**

_____ **Marital reconciliation 45**

_____ **Retirement 45**

_____ **Change in family member's health 44**

_____ **Pregnancy 40**

_____ **Sex difficulties 39**

_____ **Addition to family 39**

_____ **Business readjustment 39**

_____ **Change in financial status 38**

_____ **Death of close friend 37**

_____ **Change to a different line of work 36**

_____ **Change in number of marital arguments 35**

The Stress Response

_____ Mortgage or loan over $10,000 31

_____ Foreclosure of mortgage or loan 30

_____ Change in work responsibilities 29

_____ Trouble with in-laws 29

_____ Outstanding personal achievement 28

_____ Spouse begins or stops work 26

_____ Starting or finishing school 26

_____ Change in living conditions 25

_____ Revision of personal habits 24

_____ Trouble with boss 23

_____ Change in work hours, conditions 20

_____ Change in residence 20

_____ Change in schools 20

_____ Change in recreational habits 19

_____ Change in church activities 19

_____ Change in social activities 18

_____ Mortgage or loan under $10,000 17

_____ Change in sleeping habits 16

_____ Change in number of family gatherings 15

_____ Change in eating habits 15

_____ Vacation 13

_____ Christmas season 12

_____ Minor violations of the law 11

_____ Your Total Score

This scale shows the kind of life pressure that you are facing. Depending on your coping skills or the lack thereof, this scale can predict the likelihood that you will fall victim to a stress-related illness. The illness could be mild - frequent tension headaches, acid indigestion, loss of sleep, chronic fatigue syndrome, fibromyalgia, irritable bowel syndrome or even a life threatening illness.

LIFE STRESS SCORES

0-149 Low susceptibility to stress-related illness

150-299 Medium susceptibility to stress-related illness.

Learn and practice relaxation and stress management skills and a healthy well life style.

300 and over High susceptibility to stress-related illness

Daily practice of relaxation skills is very important for your wellness. Take care of it now before a serious illness erupts or an affliction becomes worse.

Here is an additional stress test:

Rate each question on a scale of 1 to 3

1=frequently, 2=sometimes, and 3=almost never

1. I don't have a good appetite
2. I don't get plenty of sleep (7-8 hours per night)
3. I am easily awakened by noise
4. I drink a lot of caffeinated drinks
5. I feel agitated most of the time

6. I am easily annoyed

7. I feel very impatient

8. I feel like I am always in a hurry

9. I feel fatigued

10. I feel sad

11. I feel like I can't enjoy life

12. I have trouble sleeping

13. I feel I over analyze everything

14. People tell me I over-react

15. I have a lot of health problems

16. I have a lot of headaches

17. I have a lot of stomachaches

18. I have a lot of physical pain

19. I have panic attacks

20. I worry

21. I have anxiety over something or someone almost all of the time

22. I feel angry

23. I feel fearful

24. I smoke cigarettes

25. I feel stress

If your score is 25-30, you are experiencing a great deal of stress, which may eventually compromise your job and relationships as well as your overall health and functioning; it is imperative to find a way to cope better.

If your score is 31-50, you are experiencing a moderate amount of stress, which could impair your ability to have a productive work- week and healthy relationships.

If your score is 51-75, you are functioning very well—keep up the good work!

Chapter 3

Vaccines, Germs, and Trauma

My personal journey with illness began in 1998 when constant foot pain began to plague my every step. I decided to go to a podiatrist. The podiatrist did the typical medical history on me, and proceeded to explain to me that my foot pain was a result of my running with poor shoes. He said my pain was more than likely stemming from something very common among runners called plantar fascitis, an inflammation of the fascia, the band of connective tissue connecting the heel to the edge of the toes on the bottom of the foot. The doctor assured me it was nothing to worry about, as it causes a great amount of pain and bone spurs that develop on the heel of the foot, making it painful to walk, but it was nothing serious. I believed him until the pain worsened.

Overtime I began to take measures that included cortisone shots in the bottom of my heel, a cast on my foot, acupuncture and other measures that proved unsuccessful. Finally, I visited the doctor again in January of 1999 and exclaimed, "I want surgery to cut the fascia." He was apprehensive and explained that surgery could worsen my symptoms, but that it may also be curative of my pain. Actually it was a 50/50 shot at full recovery so we decided to proceed despite his apprehension.

Before proceeding, the doctor ran a series of tests to make sure I was going to be okay for surgery. One of the tests he ran as part of a routine blood work up was a rheumatoid factor test.

Most people will have some level of rheumatoid factor in their blood. Rheumatoid factor is a type of autoantibody. An antibody is a protective protein molecule that binds specifically to an antigen. Autoantibodies, however, are antibodies that are capable of targeting one's own proteins rather than those of an outside agent, such as bacterial protein. Rheumatoid factors are autoantibodies directed against a fragment of the class of immunoglobulins known as IgG and are members of a class of proteins that become elevated in states of inflammation. Approximately seven out of 10 people who have rheumatoid arthritis have an elevated rheumatoid factor. The remaining 30 percent of the population can have an elevated rheumatoid factor for a variety of reasons. Occasionally, when no reason can be found, it is called an idiopathic false positive. The normal range for a RF test with most labs is 0 to 20 mm/hr (measuring antibodies). Anything exceeding 20 may be cause for further patient examination depending on the lab that performed the blood test. As we grow older often times our RF may increase due to age or other conditions that may include many illnesses like:

Understanding Autoimmune Disease and Stress-Related Illness

- Chronic Hepatitis
- Chronic Viral Infection
- Dermatomyositis
- Infectious Mononucleosis
- Leukemia
- Scleroderma
- Lupus
- Sjogren's Syndrome
- Endocarditis
- Tuberculosis
- Syphilis
- Sarcoidosis
- Cancer
- Vaccines

When the doctor had told me my rheumatoid factor was elevated but not enough for concern, I proceeded with surgery but in the meantime began to research what it meant to have an elevated rheumatoid factor. I had asked the doctor what it could mean and he thought nothing since my number was 30, which at that time wasn't severely elevated.

After recovery from my foot surgery, I was able to walk better, but still had some pain. I then had a long bout of increased reproductive problems as well. Some of those problems had existed for about three years prior to my foot surgery. While I was going through reproductive problems and a severely painful menses every month they had me on medications called Lupron and Danazol, just like Sara, which put me into menopause. This was a predictable result, as these drugs are commonly used for treatment of endometriosis, which after my laproscopic surgery was determined inconclusive. The Lupron and Danazol were giving me severe side effects despite what the doctor said, so I asked for a hysterectomy, which I knew had to happen. I had contemplated a hysterectomy that entire year between 1998 and 1999 and so I also decided to get Hepatitis A and B vaccinations in May of 1998, so if I needed any blood transfusions I would be less at risk for contracting Hepatitis B.

I had a hysterectomy in June of 1999. When I went for the surgery again the routine blood tests revealed that my rheumatoid factor was elevated to 80. I was beginning to experience pain throughout my body. Despite all of this, I proceeded with the procedure. The following year in the summer of 2000, I woke up one day and was unable to get out of bed, because of excruciating pain. I went to the doctor and he referred me to a rheumatologist.

The rheumatologist tested my rheumatoid factor and diagnosed me with rheumatoid arthritis, even though none of my joints were swollen or inflamed. And so my journey with autoimmune diseases and research began.

I was terrified of such a diagnosis. I wasn't able to accept it because I didn't feel as though it was conclusive. I went back to the rheumatologist and asked to have further testing to see if I had inflammation in my joints, the characteristic feature of rheumatoid arthritis. The doctor wanted to put me on a chemotherapy drug called Methotrexate in the meantime, but I declined. I returned the following week and they ran a bone scan on me through the nuclear medicine department at the local hospital. The results were unexpected. The doctor said, "everything is clear; you had a negative scan."

"I am so confused," she said echoing my sentiment. She was baffled since I was in great pain and had such a high rheumatoid factor.

I went from one specialist to another, none of whom could give me either relief from pain, or questions. The doctors were baffled. Some diagnosed fibromyalgia, while others thought cancer, and others guessed lupus. The more doctors I went to the more diagnoses I seemed to have acquired, but none with any conclusive evidence. Meanwhile I was barely able to move or even feed myself. The dilemma and the pain continued throughout the summer. I slowly began walking, then swimming and recovered much to the relief of my family and friends. However, the question still loomed what happened and why the high rheumatoid factor? Did I have a strange form of rheumatoid that suddenly went into remission? These questions were yet to be answered.

At the time of being bedridden, I had stopped being a journalist and started teaching. I then returned to college a year later to get a graduate degree in psychology with an emphasis in psychoneuroimmunology. Through this new study that concentrated on the mind-body connection of illness, I felt I might gain a better knowledge of illness.

I continued research on autoimmune diseases since I felt a great connection to these illnesses. I started doing more hours of research than I had already done and extensive interviews with researchers and doctors across the country to uncover the mystery of myself and possibly some of the mysteries behind autoimmune illnesses.

Vaccines

In looking back at that original list of possible explanations that could cause an elevated rheumatoid factor, one in particular struck me—vaccines. I began to think back to all the vaccinations I had throughout my life. I had received all of the standard childhood vaccines that included: mumps, measles, and rubella. I also had realized I received a tetanus shot as an adolescent. And occasionally I had received influenza vaccinations. Other recent vaccinations I had received included Hepatitis A and B. It was these vaccinations that piqued my interest the most as they had been administered to me so closely to the elevated rheumatoid factor and then a year and a half later widespread pain started. I wondered if these series of vaccinations, which are generally taken as a series of three for Hepatitis B and a series of two for Hepatitis A, were related.

I found several dozen research articles on vaccines, while I also visited with a specialist and researcher from a nearby medical school who was working on the same hunch. We communicated on many occasions about the relationship between vaccines and the development of autoimmune disease.

A greater confirmation of my hypothesis would begin in France. Almost half of France's 25 million inhabitants were vaccinated against Hepatitis B between 1991 and 1999. Several hundred cases of an acute central demyelinating event--possibly multiple sclerosis—followed these HB (Hepatitis B) vaccinations. They were reported to the pharmacovigilance unit in a Parisian hospital, and led to a modification of vaccination policy in the schools as well as initiation of several studies designed to examine the possible relationship between the vaccine and the central demyelinating events. The results of these studies failed to establish the causality of the HB vaccine. However, molecular mimicry between HB antigen(s) and one or more myelin proteins, or a non-specific activation of autoreactive lymphocytes, could constitute possible pathogenetic mechanisms for these adverse neurological events, according to the Federation of Neurology Hospital in Paris. In other words, the immunization may affect the way our immune system identifies a foreign invader.

In addition to this study conducted at the hospital, an additional report was released by the Department of Rheumatology at Dijon University Hospital where a questionnaire sent to nine French hospitals. Criteria for entry were rheumatic complaints of one week's duration or more, occurrence during the two months following Hepatitis B vaccination, no previously diagnosed rheumatic disease and no other explanation for the complaints. The results revealed that there were observed rheumatic disease in some of these patients following the vaccination. Further, the results also revealed an exacerbation of previously diagnosed lupus erythematosus. In the end, the findings suggested the Hepatitis B vaccination might be followed by various rheumatic conditions and might trigger the onset of underlying inflammatory or autoimmune rheumatic disease. In addition, the University of Iowa Medical Center had similar findings that reflect the relationship between the development of autoimmune disease following administration of the Hepatitis B vaccine.

After much speculation about the contribution of the Hepatitis B vaccine in autoimmune disease, researchers began to speculate what other vaccines could possibly contribute to autoimmune disease. In 1996, the U.S. Court of Federal Claims had accepted a causal relationship between rubella vaccine in the U.S. and chronic joint disease with an onset between one week and six weeks after vaccine administration.

Given the amount of information and current research that has reflected concern over the relationship of vaccinations and autoimmune disease, especially in genetically susceptible individuals, it is beneficial to do a risk/benefit analysis with a physician in determining vaccination procedure with autoimmune patients.

I then speculated there was no link to my pain and the Hepatitis B vaccination because the time frame was almost a year and a half after the vaccination and my musculoskeletal symptoms. However, I wanted greater clarification of my rheumatoid factor and whether it could be related to the Hepatitis B vaccine since my factor elevated within a couple of months after receiving the remaining series of shots.

It didn't take long to find the answer. The answer was found in Taiwan where a study had been conducted to evaluate the relationship of an elevated Rheumatoid Factor and the Hepatitis B vaccine. The Department of Internal Medicine in Kaohsiung Medical College, reported that an elevated rheumatoid factor is often found in the blood of patients with non-rheumatic disease.

My medical nightmare was not put to rest since I probably didn't have an autoimmune disease and that my rheumatoid factor was elevated from receiving the Hepatitis B vaccine.

What shocked me more was that my personal physician denied the Hepatitis B vaccine being causative in elevated rheumatoid factor and continued to insist that I had an autoimmune disease despite clinical findings, which caused me fear and anxiety.

When looking at all the findings, people like Sara and Beth could certainly have reason for concern since both received a Hepatitis B vaccine followed by rheumatic or flu-like symptoms. Anyone who has autoimmune disease in their family history or has already been diagnosed with an autoimmune disease should take caution in getting certain vaccines. Doing research on specific vaccines and their long-term side effects is the best defense.

Germs

In recent years there has been much discussion among researchers about the role bacterial and viral infections play in triggering autoimmune disease. It has been theorized that multiple sclerosis could be triggered in genetically prone individuals by different bacterial and viral infections.

Understanding Autoimmune Disease and Stress-Related Illness

The University of Utah School of Medicine conducted a study indicating that although not causative, infectious agents trigger central nervous system autoimmune disease as in the case of MS. Viral infections were shown to cause exacerbations in many MS patients. This study revealed that long after viral infections had been eradicated, it still brought with it challenges to the immune system that triggered further exacerbations. It is thought by these researchers that the prime infectious agent shows molecular mimicry with self central nervous system antigens producing a triggering CNS disease.

A study conducted by William Beaumont Hospital in Michigan revealed that 100 consecutive patients admitted to the hospital with a diagnosis of exacerbated MS were evaluated for an infectious process. A control group of 55 patients carrying the diagnosis of MS but without symptoms of neurologic decline were also studied. 35 percent of patients experiencing exacerbation of their disease were identified as having a significant bacterial infection compared with 11 percent in the control group with inactive disease. When presumptive viral and bacterial infections diagnosed before admission were included, almost 50 percent of patients had an exacerbation of their disease in response to an infection. Even urinary tract infections brought about exacerbations in some patients.

As is the case with MS, rheumatoid arthritis also has infectious disease triggers, the most notable being Helicobacter pylori or h-pylori. It is been proven that complete eradication of h-pylori bacteria, a bacteria noted for causing stomach ulcers, would reduce--and in some patients eliminate-- symptoms of RA. It has been further postulated that h-pylori is the main pathogen in those with infective RA. It was also hypothesized that infection by streptococci, the bacteria that causes strep throat, may also be a trigger, however, there was not evidence to correlate the two.

Researchers also investigated the role of herpes simplex viruses (HSV) including Cytomegalovirus (CMV) and the Epstein-Barr virus (EBV) in rheumatic diseases like Lupus. In one 1998 study, researchers took 66 rheumatic patients and examined them for IgM and IgG specific antibodies to CMV, HSV-1 and 2, and EBV.

The results of this study concluded that CMV was detected in almost 80 percent of patients, EBV in 70 percent and HSV-1 in 42 percent of patients. The study revealed that out of the 66 patients, 57 percent had active EBV and 28 percent had active CMV, with a combination of active CMV and EBV infection in 50 percent. In addition, high titers of CMV and EBV antibodies correlated with such symptoms as fever, arthritis, myalgia, carditis, hepatomegalia, migrating erythematosus eruption.

A study came out of the University of Turin in Italy on rheumatic disease and lupus. The study included 60 lupus patients that were tested for CMV and EBV and parvovirus. The study revealed a strong correlation between all of these viruses and the onset of lupus. There have also been documented cases of fibromyalgia following many of these infectious agents. And a study from the University Of Pennsylvania School Of Medicine, revealed that fibromyalgia and CFS followed after an acute parvovirus B19 infection.

Trauma

A case-controlled study to determine the role of physical trauma in the onset of fibromyalgia, examined 136 FMS patients and 152 controls that completed questionnaires about any physical trauma in the six months before the onset of their symptoms. The results of the study revealed that 39 percent of FMS patients reported significant physical trauma in the six months before the onset of their disease, compared with only 24 percent of controls. In examining that study, it would be reasonable to assume that the onset of FMS is preceded by physical trauma in some cases.

Another study examined the correlation between car accidents and onset of fibromyalgia. The Department of Neurology and Rehabilitation Medicine, City Hospital, Reykjavik, Iceland, studied 38 patients with late whiplash syndrome, and with regard to their symptoms conformed to the diagnosis of fibromyalgia.

In addition to physical traumas, emotional traumas can also take a toll on our physical health. With individuals who experienced chronic stress, whether through life events or mental illness, the toll on the body was extensive. Even daily irritations can stack up to equal a lifetime of chronic stress. And the stress for individuals who face diagnoses like Beth and Norma with bi-polar disorder, are likely to experience an almost daily emotional, psychological and physiological battle that in the end is lost in the immune system. When the immune system is so chronically compromised by our stress response to all the factors discussed in this chapter, the result is devastating and often debilitating.

Lastly, it would be reasonable to assume that after looking at all the evidence and all of the individuals I interviewed including Allen, Beth, Norma and Sara that there is a very strong correlation between vaccines, germs and trauma in triggering autoimmunity especially in those who appear to be genetically susceptible.

Chapter 4
Human Behavior and Disease

In my sophomore year of journalism school, I decided if I were to understand the world in which I would be reporting, I would need to learn about other languages and other cultures. Like other college students, I didn't have the money to travel the world, so I did the next best thing—I moved into an international community close to campus.

When I moved to this community, I realized I was one of only two English-speaking people. I befriended my suitemate who helped me survive the communication barriers. I lived among many cultures and made life-long friends with those who I lived amongst. The international students were from all over Asia, which included China, India, Thailand just to name a few. There were also many from different parts of Africa and the Middle East, as well as South America and Europe. Most of my closest friends were from Asia and Africa. As I began to eat their food, learn their languages and understand their cultures, it was an educational and exciting experience. One friend from China had family who would ship foods from home. He would cook it up and we would all share the delightful food. However, the food harbored many pathogens that could make one sick. This may have contributed to my contraction of h-pylori. Because I had never traveled to China, I speculated that the stomach bacteria I contracted had to come from the food that I consumed from there. While I thought I was safe because I was in the United States. After living in the international community and contracting many various illnesses including the Epstein-Barr virus, I decided I should get my own apartment. I moved in with my close friend from Nairobi, Kenya. He had many different customs for preparing meat and other foods, so I was careful not to eat anything that I didn't prepare myself. But what I didn't think about was that he had also lived in Calcutta, India, where they customarily don't wear shoes and are more likely to carry a foot fungus or bacteria that they may not be immune to. However, I was not immune to it and used the same shower as my friend and ended up contracting the human papilloma virus on the bottom of my foot, I had later foot problems where they had to cut one inch squares out of both feet to remove the virus. It was difficult to walk for a month and my feet were cratered. My doctor at the university scolded me for not wearing flip-flops into the shower and for eating food that may have not been inspected.

    Then came the years that followed as a journalist--meeting new people and living in new places--but mistakenly revisiting some old behaviors that proved deleterious to my health. It is my goal as a result of my experiences to help others understand that they can be in control of their health.

Understanding Autoimmune Disease and Stress-Related Illness

To help understand this phenomenon of illness, this chapter examines in further detail some human behavior, which can be very deleterious to one's health. Human-to-human behavior is responsible for approximately 70 percent of disease today, according to health experts. And the remaining disease it could be argued come from animals, which is further discussed in the diet and exercise chapter.

This book has discussed many different diseases that could possibly lead to the development of autoimmune diseases and stress-related illnesses. It is important to discuss how to possibly avoid diseases that may lead to more chronic debilitating illness such as autoimmune disease and stress-related illness.

The specific illnesses that were discussed in chapter four that could lead to the development of autoimmune diseases and stress-related illnesses include: Hepatitis A and B, h-pylori, CMV, EBV, Herpes Simplex 1 and 2, and parvovirus.

This chapter will attempt to address preventive strategies to these illnesses, which could help in not triggering a more debilitating chronic illness.

Most everyone is susceptible to any or all of these illnesses. However, with some simple precautions the odds of contraction and becoming ill can be lessened through behavioral changes.

The most revolutionary discovery in keeping people healthy wasn't antibiotics or surgery or vitamins or any other remarkable medical advancement, but the simple act of hand washing. Yet many people still don't practice adequate hand washing. It takes at least 15 seconds of vigorous hand washing with soap and water to kill disease. This behavior will keep you healthier and cleaner for your lifespan.

The next way we can become sick is through eating foods that are contaminated with anything from E-coli and salmonella to h-pylori. It is hypothesized by experts that h-pylori is contracted through contaminated food and water. Be careful what you eat, whether locally or abroad and make sure everything is adequately cooked to kill any remaining bacteria.

Should you decide to travel abroad, it is recommended that you receive Hepatitis A and B vaccines depending on where in the world you will be traveling. Again analysis with your physician as to the cost/benefit to your health and the risk of contracting these illnesses should be initiated. However, every year in the United States alone, hundreds of people are stricken with Hepatitis A and/or B (Hepatitis literally means inflammation of the liver), often contracted from a restaurant that has had a Hepatitis A outbreak. Most of these outbreaks are a result of human behavior. These outbreaks can often be traced back to a food handler who inadequately washed their hands after using the bathroom and then later handled uncooked foods like salads. Most Hepatitis A is transferred via fecal- oral contamination or through direct fecal contamination of food items. This is of course very unpleasant as the symptoms can last as long as a month and cause fatigue, nausea, vomiting, loss of appetite, fever and jaundice, according to the Centers for Disease Control.

Many individuals can contract Hepatitis B through casual sexual contact with an infected partner through any bodily fluids except saliva, so knowing your partner and getting tested as well as using safe sexual practices that include condoms will help minimize the risk. In addition to safe sex practices, avoid IV drug use, as Hepatitis B is transferred via blood contaminates. The symptoms of Hepatitis B are not very different from Hepatitis A with the only distinguishing factor perhaps being severe joint pain.

Other illnesses such as the class of herpes simplex have long plagued our society and are becoming more widespread almost at epidemic proportions because of an increase in sexual partners. And most people are completely unaware of how herpes simplex is spread or even what it is. Most people who have the occasional cold sore or fever blister attribute it to a cold. This is not always the case. All cold sores/ fever blister are caused by the herpes simplex 1 virus, which is usually acquired in early childhood from an adult who has it and kisses the child spreading the virus on to them. Herpes simplex 1 is transmittable whether or not there is a current cold sore outbreak. While there is viral shedding at least three to seven times throughout a 12- month period, no one knows when these times are. Another concern with herpes simplex 1 is during oral sexual contact. There is a risk of contracting genital herpes from having oral sex with an individual who is caring the herpes simplex 1 virus. And many people never have an outbreak either genitally or orally but are carriers and can still infect their sexual partners. This obviously poses a great health risk as most individuals are unsuspecting. And herpes simplex 2, which is caused by sexual contact, usually through intercourse, is also similar in its viral shedding and asymptomatic behavior as herpes simplex 1. It is best to always have safe sex using condoms or dental dams with infected partners and the very best protection is knowledge, so a new partner should always be tested. And if the new partner tests positive for herpes simplex 1, they are not alone, as the Centers for Disease Control estimates anywhere from 60 to 80 percent of the population is infected, while approximately one in four may be infected with herpes simplex 2. If infection has occurred, the incubation period is usually from three to seven days for either of the simplexes.

There are many different types of herpes complexes and simplexes that cause everything from the chicken pox to cytomegalovirus and mononucleosis, otherwise known as the Epstein-Barr virus. EBV has received a lot of attention in many medical circles for a variety of reasons. In my research of EBV, I reviewed the relationship of it to many different illnesses namely that of chronic fatigue syndrome. While research is skeptical of the relationship, it may be better to be safe than sorry.

Most people grew up hearing about the "kissing" disease because mono, as it is commonly referred to, is transmitted mainly through saliva. Therefore, anyone kissing, sharing utensils or toothbrushes could possibly contract the virus. In addition, the virus can also be transmitted via a sneeze or anyway that infected saliva would transfer. The most common symptoms are fatigue, fever, sore throat, and swollen lymph nodes with an incubation period of anywhere from 30 to 50 days.

The next interesting herpes simplex that has appeared in research literature as to its relationship with autoimmunity and stress-related illness, is cytomegalovirus (CMV). CMV produces almost indistinguishable symptoms from mono, and usually only a blood test can discern the difference.

Lastly, another very common illness that often strikes in childhood and generally contracted in childhood is parvovirus. Parvovirus B19 as it is referred to, is an infectious disease that commonly causes a characteristic "slap" rash across the face and also can be accompanied with a rash on the trunk and limbs. This disease again is transferred communicably via saliva, sputum and nasal mucus and is contagious about a day before the rash appears.

There are numerous infectious diseases in our world today and new ones are arising such as SARS and west nile virus, mad cow disease to name a few. I am certainly not suggesting to consume your life and thoughts with the avoidance of many of theses disease in fear of contracting them and then later developing a chronic illness, I am suggesting only to use common sense and if you can prevent exposure to these disease, then it may be in your best interest to take the extra steps to protect yourself and those you love.

Chapter 5

Childhood Abuse, Neglect, and Stress-Related Illness

Childhood abuse and neglect is at epidemic proportions in our society today. As more and more women and men are out in the work force attempting to make a living, complicated by the everyday stress of modern life, our children are undoubtedly the victims of a cursory world of fast-paced and chaotic lifestyles. And with today's pressures of needing more money and more time to live, many people are turning to the streets for answers, engaging in illegal activities and dangerous past-times that affect the children who grow up in these environments. It becomes a cycle of destruction in families where money is hard to come by often leading to drug and alcohol abuse to quiet the problems, which then often leads to physically, emotionally or neglectfully abusing their own children.

Unfortunately, this pattern of abuse potentially can become generational leading to their children abusing their children and so forth. The implications of this cycle of abuse are far reaching and multifaceted both psychologically and physiologically. This cycle of abuse can lead to mental illness and chronic health problems later in life.

It is often seen that many childhood victims of abuse and violence tend to have life-long health issues in adulthood that may manifest themselves in the form of fibromyalgia, chronic fatigue, irritable bowel syndrome, autoimmune disease, high-blood pressure and possibly even cancer. How we live our lives greatly determines our destiny psychologically and physiologically and adults who were victims of childhood abuse and neglect have a much more diligent task of maintaining their health.

It is known, according to The Final Report of the National Commission on Children that psychosocial factors influence a wide range of physiological, hormonal, and biochemical responses; and psychological factors influence the natural history of many disease states. In other words, the relations of people to their society and to the people around them can influence the incidence, the prevalence, the course, and the mortality of disease. Perhaps reducing immunologic competence at a critical time may allow a mutant cell to thrive and grow.

In addition to these psychological and physical deficits, it is postulated that children who have come from violent homes with maltreatment and abuse tend to have a different development of intellectual and emotional processing. It is theorized that these children as a result of the continued abuse process, organize and process their emotions differently than their peers. These children, as a result of the abuse, become very distressed and hostile with other children, according to mental health experts. This in turn, eventually leads to a dismal outlook for forming positive social interactions of any kind later in life or even in the immediate future for these maltreated children, often leading to issues again with intimacy, isolation and recurrent health problems.

In addition, children who have been exposed to family violence have less than favorable chances of adaptive thought patterns in response to trauma and violence. This type of cognitive deficiency is multi-faceted and multi-directional physiologically, psychologically and cognitively.

These children, who are victims of violence, experience a prolonged physiological stress response, or chronic post-traumatic stress reaction, that has been linked to changes in the functioning of the HPA axis and neurotransmitters, according to scientists. Changes have been found in the levels of several neurotransmitters that have implications for behavior and coincide with symptoms characteristic of post-traumatic stress disorder (PTSD). These include elevations in adrenalin and noradrenalin; glucocorticoids like cortisol, endogeneous opiates, and dopamine; and a reduction in serotonin. Heightened adrenalin and noradrenalin creates increased heart rates and blood flow, preparing the body and muscles for quick action, "fight or flight," but also increased agitation and perhaps decreased attention deployment capacities, according to scientists.

Childhood Abuse, Neglect, and Stress-Related Illness

In this sense, the body is constantly on high alert for perceived danger, which in turn will eventually be a detriment to the individual's emotional regulation, cognitions, and overall physical health.

Thus, the prolonged threats to survival may leave the individual in a dysregulated state, where perception, cognition, emotional systems, and physiological systems are functioning atypically and permanent changes to brain structure, especially the hippocampus, are possible. This early onset of trauma to brain structures and chemistry will lead to the child turning into an adult who will be plagued by symptoms similar to PTSD with an overly sensitive nervous system, severe anxiety and depression may follow the individual through life. This again will lead to a chronic state of fight-or-flight leading to many physiological and psychological problems in the future. This speculation and supportive research are based on a study of adult PTSD victims.

This sets the child up for a lifetime of possible health problems that could further manifest into illnesses such as high-blood pressure, autoimmune disease, irritable bowel syndrome, fibromyalgia and chronic fatigue syndrome.

The Division of Rheumatology and Immunology at the University of North Carolina, Chapel Hill, reported that just as our caveman forebears were frail in the face of predatory animals, we are frail in today's society of childhood neglect or abuse, bumper-to-bumper traffic, frustration at work, and multiple daily hassles. The same neuroendocrine systems and pain regulatory mechanisms that protected early man during acute stress are still encoded in our genome but may be maladaptive in psychologically and physiologically vulnerable people faced with chronic stress.

Many patients with fibromyalgia become vulnerable people faced with chronic stress, because of the long-lasting psychological and neurophysiological effects of negative experiences in childhood. They display maladaptive coping strategies, low self-efficacy, and negative mood when confronted with the inevitable stressors of life. Psychological distress ensues, which reduces thresholds for pain perception and tolerance, which is already relatively low in women.

Further reported by the University of North Carolina, Chapel Hill, converging lines of psychological and neurobiological evidence strongly suggest that chronic stress-related blunting of the HPA, sympathetic, and other axes of the stress response, together with associated alterations in pain regulatory mechanisms may finally explain the pain and fatigue of fibromyalgia. Vulnerable people who can be classified under specific criteria as having fibromyalgia do not have a discrete disease. They are simply the most ill in a continuum of distress, chronic pain, and painful tender points in the general population.

In addition to physical abuse and neglect, sexual abuse has also been implicated in contributing to long-term health problems that later in life may manifest into fibromyalgia and chronic fatigue syndromes. A study suggesting this type of strong correlation was conducted by the Department of Physical Medicine and Rehabilitation at London Health Sciences Centre out of Ontario, Canada, suggesting that women with a history of childhood sexual abuse reported more chronic pain symptoms and utilized more health-care resources compared to individuals who were not abused.

A further study conducted by the Department of Psychiatry and Behavioral Sciences at the University of Washington in Seattle, compared fibromyalgia patients alongside rheumatoid arthritis patients through interviewing individuals on sexual, physical, and emotional victimization histories, as well as reports of the severity of each of these victimizations also revealed similar results.

The study found that compared with the patients with rheumatoid arthritis, those with fibromyalgia had significantly higher lifetime prevalence rates of all forms of victimization, both adult and childhood. Trauma severity was correlated significantly with measures of physical disability, psychiatric distress, illness adjustment, personality, and quality of sleep in patients with fibromyalgia, but not in those with rheumatoid arthritis.

In conclusion of this study, it is reasonable to correlate that fibromyalgia seems to be associated with increased risk of victimization, particularly adult physical abuse. Sexual, physical, and emotional trauma may be important factors in the development and maintenance of this disorder and its associated disability in many patients.

In addition, a study was conducted by the Department of Psychosomatic Rehabilitation at the University of Belgium, which studied the correlations of victimization in fibromyalgia and CFS patients when compared to patients suffering from rheumatoid arthritis and multiple sclerosis that further made concrete correlations for those suffering from fibromyalgia and/or CFS as having experienced long-term victimization in the areas of emotional, sexual and physical abuse. CFS and FMS patients showed significantly high prevalence's of emotional neglect and physical abuse. Their primary family of origin (biological mother and father) and partners were the most frequent perpetrators. With the exception of sexual abuse, victimization was more severe in the CFS and FMS patients, and absolutely no differences were found between the RA and MS patients.

Therefore, we can conclude that chronic stress directly related to physical, sexual and even emotional abuse, plays a pivotal role in the development of CFS and FMS, especially for women in our society who are experiencing significantly more severe, on-going physical, emotional and sexual abuse than men since in most cases the overwhelming perpetrators are men. This naturally leads to more long-term implications for women, which inevitably has long-term therapeutic implications and possible psychosocial interventions that will need to be further investigated and implemented.

Part II:
Autoimmune Disease and Stress-Related Survival

Chapter 6

Diagnosis and Treatments for Healthcare Professionals

Autoimmune and stress-related illnesses are by far, according to medical doctors, the most difficult class of illnesses to diagnose and treat. Most medical doctors and scientists would agree that these classes of disease are the most elusive and unpredictable of any disease in the modern world. Most experts would also agree that we know little to nothing about autoimmune disease and stress-related illness. While as researchers and scientists, we can postulate as to what the possible causes are, it is still a mystery as to why one person over another in the same set of circumstances may not develop the same disease state. These diseases are also so unpredictable in their course of development and exacerbations that it leaves the patient feeling utterly frightened and unsettled even when current symptoms of the disease are not presenting themselves.

Furthermore, these diseases on average take approximately five years to diagnose properly, because the course of these diseases is so unpredictable. This leaves the patient and the practitioner frustrated and helpless in figuring out a solution. This leads to greater anxiety for the patient, which can leave them feeling worse. Often time's patients are diagnosed with all of the autoimmune diseases and stress-related illnesses before a concrete diagnosis can be established. One reason for this cross-over affect, is many of the autoimmune diseases and stress-related illnesses often exhibit similar symptoms in the beginning, making it difficult for the patient or the practitioner to distinguish one from the other until comprehensive diagnostic tests are performed, as well as a comprehensive review of the patient's symptoms and clinical presentations. Together with all of these diagnostic tools and some time on everyone's side, a more accurate diagnosis will emerge.

However, many of these diagnostic tools are not always accurate and can be very costly to the patient adding more stress to their lives. These tools are all physicians have to attempt a diagnosis. In addition to all the diagnostic tools, there are just as many treatment options that can be equally confusing, and costly to the patient. Although necessary for the patient in many cases, the overall cost on their health and pocket book must be weighed with their physician.

Since the early 21st Century, there have been strides in the treatment of many of these diseases with better success than in previous years. However, with other illnesses like fibromyalgia and chronic fatigue syndrome there has yet to be a concrete blood test or proven effective treatment.

Fibromyalgia Diagnosis and Treatment:

To start, an illness like fibromyalgia can mimic many other illnesses that can have similar symptoms. For this reason it is difficult to diagnose these individuals. The standard symptoms of fibromyalgia are a flu-like syndrome that manifests itself in severe aching throughout the body with specific tender points that are severely sensitive. According to the American College of Rheumatology, there are 18 specific tender points that occur with fibromyalgia. Because all but a few points occur from the waist up along the lower lumbar and upper cervical spine as well as around the clavicle, it seems natural to assume that car accidents play a role in triggering pain in these regions, which can become chronic when combined with other factors. This possibly leading to what is now termed fibromyalgia syndrome.

However, even after the patient has presented to the doctor these clinical symptoms, there is still no concrete way of proving the patient actually has this syndrome. It essentially becomes a diagnosis of exclusion. After the doctor has run up a bill costing several thousands of dollars and several arm pricks later, the doctor finally comes to the conclusion that this person may have fibromyalgia.

However, in the medical establishment many doctors do not believe that this syndrome exists. They believe it is a compilation of symptoms playing in concert with many other issues the patient might have, like mental illness, ranging from bi-polar disorder to a chronic-stress response due to trauma. However, they all agree no matter what the cause, the patient is experiencing illness and pain that needs to be treated. And this is where it becomes extremely tricky. This is why it is very important to find a doctor who has the same perspective on fibromyalgia as the patient otherwise the treatment might be very different.

For example, if a doctor believes this is strictly a somatic mental illness of hypochondria or other somatic mental illness, then perhaps the patient will be referred to a psychiatrist who will prescribe medication to treat the mental disorder, which may not be an effective treatment for the patient's fibromyalgia syndrome. Or perhaps the doctor himself decides to prescribe psychotropic medications for the patient. Or the doctor may believe that fibromyalgia is the result of physical trauma to the body like a car accident or on-going physical abuse, in which they may prescribe pain-killers, muscle relaxers and hot/cold treatments or ultrasound therapy. Then there are the doctors of osteopathy that take a more holistic approach to medicine, and they may suggest a skeletal adjustment, massage therapy and acupuncture. And should the patient choose to go to a naturopathic doctor, they may prescribe anything from herbs and exercise, to having the patient stand on their head with magnets.

Because of the almost thousands of explanations by doctors and researchers as to the cause of fibromyalgia and the wide range of treatments it is imperative to become educated on all fronts and try what works best and provides the most relief.

In addition to all the possible causes that have been discussed in previous chapters, researchers are definitely suspecting that this illness is more neurologically mediated through the immune system and not a single pain event that causes inflammation or swelling. Because fibromyalgia patients don't experience inflammation and swelling, it is baffling as to why doctors will prescribe anti-inflammatory medications (NSAIDs) with no success. Also doctors tend to prescribe muscle relaxants like Flexeril, which again only have moderate success at best.

However, several classes of drugs have proven somewhat helpful in the treatment of pain symptoms. In June 2007, Lyrica became the first medication to be FDA approved as a fibromyalgia treatment. In clinical trials, people with FMS showed significant improvement in pain, sleep, fatigue and quality of life. In addition to Lyrica, the FDA approved Cymbalta and Savalla as fibromyalgia treatments. These drugs are classified as SNRI's, or serotonin-norepinephrine reuptake inhibitors. Other drugs used are the Selective Serotonin Reuptake Inhibitors (SSRI's) class of anti-depressant drugs that can include everything from Prozac to Zoloft. Also tricyclic antidepressants like Trazadone have had some level of success because these antidepressants have an effect on sleep patterns.

Diagnosis and Treatments for Healthcare Professionals

    This lends even more evidence that this illness could be part of a chronic stress response that is neurologically mediated through the immune system causing a vicious cycle of illness. Another avenue that has certainly been explored with moderate success for these patients is swimming and walking in a warm pool. This may serve at least a couple of purposes. First, it can help to raise serotonin levels naturally, which can provide pain relief, and the buoyancy of the water can provide a soothing relief to achy joints and muscles.

    Furthermore, many patients have found great relief with massage therapy and meditation for pain reduction and better sleep, since many fibro patients suffer from lack of deep sleep, which provides the body with much needed repair of organs and tissues. Other patients have found relief with basic stretching exercises and yoga.

    Another interesting avenue of treatment is hormone replacement, but not with estrogen—it is with male sex hormones that include everything from testosterone to progesterone. Many women have low levels of testosterone and may benefit greatly from taking supplemental testosterone and progesterone (which also turns into testosterone in the body). Also another side benefit to taking these hormones, which should only be taken as a topical, natural ointment rubbed on the skin, is the great benefits to women's bones. According to medical experts, progesterone and testosterone when used together can protect women from developing osteoporosis without the harmful side effects of traditional oral hormone replacement therapies like Premarin. A problem with giving fibromyalgia patients a plethora of drugs is they may not be properly digesting and absorbing these medications, therefore they are not getting the full benefits. Also these male sex hormones can help take some stress off the adrenal glands. This will allow less cortisol to be released, which lessens pain and bone loss, and also provides the patient with more energy and less chance of anxiety because less stress hormones are being released. And the immune system will also thank you for taking some of the burden from the stress response.

Often time's people who have stress-related illness also have many accompanied functional illnesses like irritable bowel syndrome and often these individuals may have an autoimmune disease like ulcerative colitis, which doesn't allow nutrients to absorb into the body properly. This negates the benefits of many drugs.

Chronic Fatigue Syndrome Diagnosis and Treatment:

Much like fibromyalgia, chronic fatigue syndrome is also incredibly elusive for both the patient and their doctors. As discussed in previous chapters, many viruses and traumas have been implicated as possible causative factors in the development of CFS. As with many things in medicine, nothing has proven conclusive. And because it is hard to understand all the features and causes of CFS, it is also hard to diagnose and treat. Much like fibromyalgia, CFS also doesn't have lab tests to prove its existence, so again it is often a diagnosis of exclusion.

And similarly, fibromyalgia, and CFS, have many of the same treatment options aimed at helping with pain and sleep. Those suffering from chronic fatigue syndrome are experiencing unrelenting exhaustion that can't be relieved by any amount of sleep. Therefore, it is important to focus on attempting to help the person get better sleep, not necessarily more sleep. This can be achieved often times by using anti-depressant medication that will help sleep and pain. An exercise regime that isn't too strenuous, aimed at building stamina may be helpful.
If all else fails, Provigil can be used. A study presented at the 2006 annual meeting of the American Psychiatric Association in Toronto showed promising results indicating that modafinil (Provigil) could reduce some of the fibromyalgia-related fatigue and CFS.

The study, presented by Dr. Thomas L. Schwartz and Dr. Susan M. Chlebowski of the State University of New York in Syracuse, reviewed 98 fibromyalgia/ CFS patients who were being treated with modafinil. Their dosages ranged from 200 to 400 mg./day. On average, two-thirds of the patients experienced a 50 percent reduction in fatigue levels

Again, meditation and herbs may prove helpful as well. As with FMS, the introduction of topical progesterone and testosterone may again help with the cycle of adrenal burnout, which may lead to CFS. By taking the burden off of the adrenals, these hormones have proven effective in providing more energy, lessening depression and increasing sex drive for those with both FMS and CFS.

Rheumatoid Arthritis Diagnosis and Treatment:
Although very difficult to diagnose and treat, RA has more distinguishable diagnostic tools like lab tests, x-rays, bone scans, and a host of other diagnostic tools. Often in the beginning it is difficult to discern RA from illnesses such as lupus, since many of the same clinical symptoms can appear early in the course of both diseases, like swelling and inflammation of joints.

However, there are diagnostic tools used specifically to discern the difference. The first type of diagnostic tool—the rheumatoid factor blood test can alert the doctor that there is an autoantibody reaction possibly occurring. However, as discussed in previous chapters, an elevated rheumatoid factor can be elevated for a variety of reasons or for no reason at all, so this test isn't exactly specific to rheumatoid arthritis, but can be helpful when combined with many other diagnostic measures.

The next test a doctor may order if there is an elevated rheumatoid factor, is the erythrocyte sedimentation rate (ESR) test. This test measures the amount of inflammation the body is experiencing. However, like the rheumatoid factor test, it is not specific to inflammation caused by rheumatoid. For instance, if a person is sick with a severe respiratory infection or some type of injury they may have an elevated ESR.

The next test that has more accuracy is the C-reactive protein test (CRP). This test can be used during an acute flair up much like the ESR; both tests have different attributes of measurement. A rule of thumb is to give both tests to cover all bases.

Another test that is less widely used by rheumatologists, is the HLA-DR4 genetic marker test. Half to three-fourths of patients with RA carry the HLA-DR4 marker (HLA is the human leukocyte antigen), but some fifty percent of the population may also carry HLA-DR4 and never develop RA, so again it isn't very specific. HLA is, however, being widely investigated by researchers much like the CTLA4 marker in the development autoimmune disease. HLA is considered by researchers to be a very important factor in the immune response. Researchers believe that the gene CTLA4 may contribute to autoimmune disease if it mutates causing an increase in susceptibility to a variety of autoimmune disorders.

Other blood tests that are controversial and not specific or sensitive include: antifilagrin antibody, antiperinuclear factor, and antikeratin antibody tests.

Understanding Autoimmune Disease and Stress-Related Illness

The remaining diagnostic tools are the basic x-ray to determine joint destruction and deformity, and the bone scan, which uses nuclear medicine to identify "hot spots" of inflammation in joints throughout the body. An individual having a bone scan for this purpose, may light up like a Christmas tree on the scan, and if there are no "hot spots" of inflammation the diagnostician may need to look to another diagnosis depending on other observations.

Depending on the course and the severity of the disease, many different treatments will need to be explored. These treatments include many varieties of drugs aimed at stopping inflammation and joint destruction, as well as pain control and improved quality of life.

The first class of drugs used for pain and inflammation are anti-inflammatory medications like aspirin or ibuprofen. These medications work specifically on reducing circulating prostaglandins, which are hormones that contribute to the inflammatory process in the body. Another class of drugs used in the fight to reduce inflammation and pain are the corticosteroids. These drugs are often used in combination with other medications. It is also common practice to formulate a drug cocktail that could include many drug classes to provide maximum benefit to the patient.

The classes of drugs that have the least amount of side-effects that are commonly used in treating RA, are the class of anti-inflammatory drugs called Cox-2 inhibitors. These drugs also inhibit prostaglandins, and are touted by pharmaceutical companies as less damaging to the stomach lining than traditional anti-flammatory drugs like ibuprofen or aspirin, which may produce stomach ulcerations and gastrointestinal upset.

Furthermore, another drug class being investigated more thoroughly is the use of antibiotics like Minocycline, and Sulfasalazine to treat inflammation. Medications like Minocycline were used in the treatment of acne, but have recently showed promise in slowing the inflammatory process.

Some of the medications that help alleviate joint deformity, pain and mobilization include everything from anti-inflammatory medications, to a newer class of drugs called DMARDs, which stands for disease-modifying anti-rheumatic drugs, which work specifically to depress areas of the immune system that cause inflammation. The DMARDs are used usually after aspirin prednisone and ibuprofen have failed to halt disease progression. According to the National Institute of Health and the Arthritis Foundation these are some of the drugs referred to as DMARDs:

- *Methotrexate—side effects may include:* can adversely affect kidneys and liver; also may cause stomach upset and flu-like symptoms, and mouth sores—some of these side effects can be reduced by using in conjunction the vitamin folate

- *Arava—side effects may include:*
  diarrhea, hair loss and rash

- **Leflunomide--** *side effects may include:*
  gastrointestinal (GI) symptoms, skin rashes, and reversible hair loss, Leflunomide should not be taken by people with active infections, or who are pregnant or nursing. Because studies have shown that Leflunomide can cause birth defects in animals, so women of childbearing age must take exceptional care to prevent pregnancy while taking the drug

- **Imuran--** *side effects may include:*
  As an immunosuppresant like all DMARDs, damage to liver and kidneys; severe infections may also occur

- *Plaqueni—side effects may include:*
  this drug was originally used for the treatment of malaria and patients need to have eye exams to monitor retinal damage

- *Cuprimine--side effects may include:*

GI upset, hives, fever, weakness, swollen glands, joint pain, kidney and liver problems

- *Cytoxan--side effects may include:*
  GI upset, more susceptible to infection, weakness and tiredness

- *Sandimmune—side effects may include:*
  GI upset, increased susceptibility to infection, tender gums, high blood pressure, kidney problems, trembling hands

- *Ridaura-- side effects may include:*
  increase sun sensitivity, GI upset, mouth sores, skin rash and kidney problems

- *Gold Sodium--side effects may include*:
  increased sun sensitivity, metallic taste, initial increased joint pain, mouth soreness

The DMARDs in general cause an increased risk of infection due to their effects on the immune system, and most cause an increase in GI upset, so use with caution under the supervision of a medical doctor.

Another class of drugs on the market is the BRMs or biologic response modifiers. These drugs work by targeting specific parts of the immune system blocking the tumor necrosis factor (TNF), a chemical that is specific to the inflammatory process of the immune system. The main drugs included in this class are Enbrel and Remicade both causing much of the same side effects of GI upset and an increased risk of infection.

Multiple Sclerosis Diagnosis and Treatment:

Diagnosing and treating MS can be as difficult as all other autoimmune illnesses. For some, MS can start out as insidious as fatigue or depression. While others begin to experience problems with vision that can include anything from blurred to double vision, still others may experience many neurological deficits like numbness, weakness or tingling in various parts of the body like a hand or foot. All of these can wax and wane during the course of attempting to clinically diagnose a patient based on their symptoms. And because many of these symptoms can be other illnesses other than MS, it is especially important to pursue a more in-depth approach with a neurologist if MS is suspected.

After deciding that MS could be causing these problems, a neurologist, who specializes in the treatment of MS and other neurological diseases, will generally order either an MRI (Magnetic Resonance Imaging) or a spinal tap to examine cerebrospinal fluid.

In recent years, the MRI has proved to be the gold standard of diagnosing MS. Because the MRI provides an in-depth view of the spine and brain, it enables radiologists to look at tissues in the brain that could be affected by lesions caused by the demyelination that MS causes.

Furthermore, taking a spinal tap can also help in piecing together a diagnosis. The spinal fluid in many MS patients generally has more white blood cells and more protein than normal. And certain antibodies in the fluid may also be present. Currently, researchers are further investigating the genetic links to MS and other autoimmune disease through the HLA marker also found in RA patients. This particular marker for MS patients is specific to the HLA-DR2, which like all the HLA markers are known to be an important factor in the immune response. However, testing for this is neither routine nor available in doctor's offices, and is again not conclusive in and of itself for MS. It is merely another possible factor in the development of the disease.

Treatment for MS patients has improved greatly over the last 10 years with the introduction of Interferon, which is produced naturally by the immune system. In its natural state in the body, Interferon provides protection against virus invasion and inhibits viral growth, but for MS patients it helps limit exacerbations of the disease.

Understanding Autoimmune Disease and Stress-Related Illness

The following list of current treatments for MS patients that are disease modifying (*provided by National MS Society*)

- *Avonex-- side effects may include:*

  Flu-like symptoms following injection, which lessen over time for many people. Rare: mild anemia, elevated liver enzymes.

- *Betaseron-- side effects may include:*

  Flu-like symptoms following injection, which lessen over time for many. Injection site reactions, about 5% of which need medical attention. In rare cases: elevated liver enzymes, low white blood cell counts.

- *Copaxone—side effects may include:*

  Injection site reactions. In rare cases: a reaction immediately after injection, which includes anxiety, chest tightness, shortness of breath, and flushing. This lasts 15-30 minutes and has no known long-term effects.

- *Novantrone—side effects may include:*

  nausea, mild hair loss, urinary tract infections, and menstrual disorders including amenorrhea (absence of menstrual period, in 25% of females). Novantrone can increase the risk for infection, because it decreases the number of protective white blood cells.

- *Rebif—side effects may include:*

  Flu-like symptoms following injection, which lessen over time for many; injection site reactions; less common: Abnormalities of liver function and decreases in red or white blood cell counts.

In between exacerbations corticosteroids are also used to ease symptoms in conjunction with the above DMARDs. The drug Solu-medrol (methylprednisolone) is commonly used for this purpose with possible side effects including susceptibility to infection, GI upset, rash, bloating, weight gain and weakness.

Lupus Diagnosis and Treatment:

According to the National Institutes of Health Division of Arthritis and Musculoskeletal and Skin Diseases (NIAMS), diagnosing lupus can be difficult. It may take months or even

Understanding Autoimmune Disease and Stress-Related Illness

years for doctors to piece together the symptoms to diagnose this complex disease accurately. Often times coming up with an accurate diagnosis is highly dependant upon what the patient reports. Giving the doctor a complete, accurate medical history (for example, what health problems you have had and for how long) is critical to the process of diagnosis. This information, along with a physical examination and the results of laboratory tests, helps the doctor consider other diseases that may mimic lupus, or determine if the patient truly has the disease, according to the NIAMS. Like all the other autoimmune disorders, no single test can determine whether a person has lupus, but several laboratory tests may help the doctor to make a diagnosis.

Often, the most useful tests identify certain autoantibodies often present in the blood of people with lupus. For example, the antinuclear antibody (ANA) test is commonly used to look for autoantibodies that react against components of the nucleus, or "command center," of the patient's own cells, according to the NIAMS. Most people with lupus test positive for ANA; however, there are a number of other causes of a positive ANA besides lupus, including infections, other rheumatic or immune diseases, and occasionally as a finding in normal healthy adults. The ANA test simply provides another clue for the doctor to consider in making a diagnosis. In addition, there are blood tests for individual types of autoantibodies that are more specific to people with lupus, although not all people with lupus test positive for these and not all people with these antibodies have lupus. These antibodies include anti-DNA, anti-Sm, anti-RNP, anti-Ro (SSA), and anti-La (SSB), according to NIAMS. There is a genetic link to the HLA marker in lupus patients. Many of these patients often have an elevated HLA-B8 marker. However, testing for this is neither routine nor available in doctor's offices, and is again not conclusive for lupus. It is merely another possible factor in the development of the disease.

After many laboratory tests have been exhausted, the doctor may order a biopsy of the skin or kidneys if those body systems are affected. Some doctors may order a syphilis test or a test for anticardiolipin antibody. A positive test does not mean that a patient has syphilis; however, the presence of this antibody may increase the risk of blood clotting and can increase the risk of miscarriages in pregnant women with lupus. These tests serve as tools to give the doctor clues and information in making a diagnosis. The doctor will look at the entire picture--medical history, symptoms, and test results--to determine if a person has lupus.

According to the NIAMS, other laboratory tests are used to monitor the progress of the disease once it has been diagnosed. A complete blood count, urinalysis, blood chemistries, and the ESR test can provide valuable information. Another common test measures the blood level of a group of substances called

Understanding Autoimmune Disease and Stress-Related Illness

complement. People with lupus often have increased ESRs and low complement levels, especially during flares of the disease.

According to the NIAMS, the range and effectiveness of treatments for lupus have increased dramatically, giving doctors more choices in how to treat the disease. Once lupus has been diagnosed, the doctor will develop a treatment plan based on the patient's age, sex, health, symptoms, and lifestyle. Treatment plans are tailored to the individual's needs and may change over time. In developing a treatment plan, the doctor has several goals: to prevent flares, to treat them when they do occur, and to minimize organ damage and complications. The doctor and patient should re-evaluate the plan regularly to ensure that it is as effective as possible.

Several types of drugs are used to treat lupus (information obtained from the NIAMS)

The treatment the doctor chooses is based on the patient's individual symptoms and needs. For people with joint or chest pain or fever, drugs that decrease inflammation are used. Anti-inflammatory medications may be used alone or in combination with other types of drugs to control pain, swelling, and fever. Common side effects of NSAIDs, including those available over the counter, can include stomach upset, heartburn, diarrhea, and fluid retention. Some patients with lupus also develop liver and kidney inflammation while taking NSAIDs, making it especially important to stay in close contact with the doctor while taking these medications. And anti-inflammatory drugs like the COX-2 inhibitors are also used, however, patients should use extreme caution with this class of anti-inflammatory medications as they have not been extensively studied in patients with lupus. Furthermore, the FDA has not approved COX-2 inhibitors for use specifically in lupus.

Furthermore, another class of drugs used to treat lupus with some success has been the anti-malaria drugs. A common anti-malaria drug used to treat lupus is hydroxychloroquine (Plaquenil). It may be used alone or in combination with other drugs and generally is used to treat fatigue, joint pain, skin rashes, and inflammation of the lungs. Clinical studies have found that continuous treatment with anti-malaria drugs may prevent flares from recurring. Side effects of anti-malaria drugs can include stomach upset and, extremely rarely, damage to the retina of the eye. The mainstay of lupus treatment, however, involves the use of corticosteroid hormones, such as prednisone (Deltasone), hydrocortisone, methylprednisolone (Medrol), and dexamethasone (Decadron, Hexadrol). Corticosteroids are related to cortisol, which is a natural anti-inflammatory hormone. They work by rapidly suppressing inflammation. Corticosteroids can be given by mouth, in creams applied to the skin, or by injection. Because they are potent drugs, the doctor will seek the lowest dose with the greatest benefit. Short-term side effects of corticosteroids include swelling, increased appetite, weight gain, and emotional instability. These side effects generally stop when the drug is stopped. It can be dangerous to stop taking corticosteroids suddenly, so it is very important that the doctor and patient work together in changing the corticosteroid dose.

Long-term side effects of corticosteroids can include stretch marks on the skin, excessive hair growth, weakened or damaged bones (osteoporosis and osteonecrosis), high blood pressure, damage to the arteries, high blood sugar, infections, and cataracts. Typically, the higher the dose of prolonged corticosteroids, the more severe the side effects. Also, the longer they are taken, the greater the risk of side effects. Researchers are working to develop alternative strategies to limit or offset the use of corticosteroids. For example, corticosteroids may be used in combination with other, less potent drugs, or the doctor may try to slowly decrease the dose once the disease is under control. People with lupus who are using corticosteroids should talk to their doctors about taking supplemental calcium and vitamin D or other drugs to reduce the risk of osteoporosis.

Patients who have many body systems affected by the disease may receive intravenous gamma globulin (Gammagard S/D), a blood protein that increases immunity and helps fight infection. Gamma globulin also may be used to control acute bleeding in patients with thrombocytopenia or to prepare a person with lupus for surgery. Also DMARDs like methotrexate may also be used in combination with many of these other medications.

However, when many of these drugs have failed to halt the progression of the disease process and inflammation, Cyclophosphamide and Azathioprine may be used as a last line of defense to protect against possible organ destruction.

Cyclophosphamide is a drug used in the treatment of various cancers, and it is used to treat patients with lupus when major organs, such as the kidneys, are affected. It is also used to treat severe inflammation that has not responded to corticosteroids. In lupus, the immune system is too active. Cyclophosphamide slows down the immune system so that disease activity can be reduced.

Side effects may include:
nausea, vomiting, loss of appetite, mouth ulcers, fatigue, temporary hair loss, unusual bleeding or blood in the urine, shortness of breath, loss of menstrual periods, impotence, sterility, or signs of infection (such as increased temperature, sore throat, or flu symptoms).

Azathioprine is a drug that acts to suppress the work of the immune system as well. It is used mainly in organ transplantation to prevent the body from rejecting the new organ. The drug is also used in patients with lupus who have damage to their kidneys or other organs, muscle inflammation, or advanced arthritis. Azathioprine helps to reduce symptoms and damage to the affected organs. It can also help achieve a remission of the disease.

Side effects may include:

stomach upset, nausea, vomiting, abdominal pain, mouth ulcers, darkened urine, pale stools, jaundice (yellowing of the skin or white portion of the eyes), unusual bleeding or bruising, signs of infection (such as chills, fever, sore throat, or fatigue

Chapter 7

Feeling Better: A Maintenance Plan

Alternative Treatments

Acupuncture

Acupuncture, has been used for many thousands of years in some form or another in China, and has had therapeutic results for many diseases, such as arthritis. Arthritis sufferers experienced some degree of pain relief from the use of acupuncture. Acupuncture uses very fine, small needles inserted at intricate parts on the body to deliver qi (Chee) to balance the body and provide pain relief. Rheumatoid patients may also find some benefit from this practice.

In the treatment of trigger points for persons experiencing pain, dry needling is an invasive procedure in which an acupuncture needle is inserted into the skin and muscle directly at a myofascial trigger point. A myofascial trigger point consists of multiple contraction knots, which are related to the production and maintenance of the pain cycle. Proper dry needling of a myofascial trigger point will elicit a local twitch response (LTR), which is an involuntary spinal cord reflex in which the muscle fibers in the taut band of muscle contract. The LTR indicates the proper placement of the needle in a trigger point. Research has indicated that dry needling that elicits LTRs improves treatment outcomes and can be effective for pain relief related to trauma.

Homeopathic and Naturopathic Remedies

Bee and snake venom along with other homeopathic remedies have been used for the treatment of RA. Many alternative practitioners taught the benefits of venom in reducing the pain and symptoms of RA. However, most medical doctors are skeptical of this practice, and warn about its dangers of possible death and toxicity to the patient. Venom therapies utilize the body's natural tendency toward health by gently challenging the immune systems to correct the health imbalance. The use of essential oils, diet, exercise, flower remedies, and herbal or other elemental tinctures to stimulate the body to heal is an ancient technique. A variety of techniques to stimulate healing, are also assets in treating depression, anxiety, allergies, and some addictions. The treatments are generally gentle and well tolerated. Clients are urged to utilize practitioners with experience in treating their specific illness.

Ayurvedic Medicine

Ayurvedic Medicines, which originated in India thousands of years ago, may provide some relief to RA sufferers. For instnce, researchers reported to the American College of Rheumatology that combining ginger, turmeric, and frankincense provided significant and sustained pain relief, reduction in the number and severity of swollen joints and reduced stiffness.

There are dozens of alternative therapies available to treat autoimmune diseases, chronic pain, and stress related illnesses. Among the more commonly available—acupuncture, chiropractic, massage, yoga, naturopathy, homeopathy, osteopathy, and meditation—I have found each of these to be a valued resource.

Aromatherapy

Aromatherapy can also be helpful during a hot bath or during meditation to help with relaxation and enliven the senses.

Magnetic Therapy

Magnetic Therapy has also been investigated by practitioners for pain relief in RA patients; however, its efficacy has yet to be established.

Special Note: *(In addition to many hospitals and universities sponsoring clinical trials, it is also important for the consumer to be aware of the role of biotechnology companies. Biotech firms provide cutting-edge research and clinical trials and most can be found on-line by entering the specific name of the disease and the word "biotechnology labs" on google.com or other search engines)*

Massage and Yoga

Massage and Yoga offer stress-relief and body centering exercise practiced for centuries by Asian cultures to restore balance and promote relaxation and mind cleansing.

These treatment modalities have a long tradition in treating bodily and emotional ills. I recommend them to clients with or without health challenges. Both are helpful in treating arthritis, lupus, chronic pain, depression, fibromyalgia and chronic fatigue syndrome. Even diabetes may respond to massage and yoga, as they relax the individual and help restore circulation in the extremities. I always caution clients to avoid deep muscle massage when first experiencing this resource. A gentle massage may be more useful at first to assist the body's immune system by using easy, regular stimulation of the muscles and joints. We do not want to shock the body, but encourage it to heal.

Clients who have been ill for some time find that exercise is no longer part of their daily routine. Urge them to gradually include light exercise in their daily activities. Some examples of exercises that can be done with low impact on sore joints are walking, swimming, stretching, stationary cycling, Pilates, health balls, and light weight training. Deep breathing exercises may be the first physical challenge some clients are able to maintain.

Some clients find exercise to be boring. Having a series of rewards to encourage continued exercise can also stimulate more interest in the activity as well as having exercise buddies, reading while cycling on a stationary bike, or listening to music or a book on tape during the routine.

Suggest that individuals look into taking classes for the elderly, which are usually low impact, such as water aerobics, and progress from there when ready. Advise against heavy exercise if one has not been in the habit for some time. Do not subscribe to the idea that no pain produces no gain. It is the opposite in these cases, as autoimmune illnesses are generally by harsh challenges to the physiology.

If discomfort does occur, the use of hot tubs, saunas, and warm compresses or ice bags to relieve some musculoskeletal strains is also advised if the client's physician so approves. It is important to start with a very light routine and increase gradually.

Exercise should also include proper hydration. However, even when not exercising, I encourage clients to drink water. The formula used at high altitude (one mile) is to take your body weight, divide it in half, drink that many ounces of water per day (for example, if you weigh 150 pounds, you should drink 75 ounces of water per day), not to exceed one gallon. Some athletes can drink more water, but they also add salt and enzyme restorative drinks to their diet. While it is essential to drink sufficient water, it is also important to augment water with salts when needed. Water is the basis for our body's chemistry, but so are enzymes and salts. If one is ill, drinking fluids can help encourage healing by flushing wastes from the body, assisting in digestion, and providing the basis for the myriad chemical reactions in our cells.

Osteopathy

This branch of medical treatment utilizes numerous alternative therapies. Osteopaths are often trained in nutrition, chiropractic, and physical therapy, in addition to allopathic medicine. They can be of great use in establishing a holistic health regimen. While I have not been able to refer to their services frequently, when I have referred clients with allergies, arthritis, chronic pain, and stress related disorders, they have been treated well and received much relief.

Trigger-Point Injections as a Fibromyalgia Treatment

A trigger point differs from the 18 tender points used to diagnose fibromyalgia. Trigger points are tight, ropy bands of muscle that form when a muscle does not relax properly. They're often formed as a result of physical trauma, but doctors don't yet understand why some people develop them while others do not. The trigger point can irritate or trap nerves and cause what's called referred pain, which is pain felt elsewhere along the nerve. Frequently, you can feel a trigger point just below the skin, and if you push on it you could cause an involuntary twitch.

Trigger-point injections (TPIs) are used to treat these extremely painful areas. The doctor inserts a small needle directly into the trigger point and injects a local anesthetic such as lidocaine or procaine. (Doctors frequently use corticosteroids as well, but these drugs are not recommended for FMS patients.) The injection can cause a twitch or pain that last for up to a few minutes. Patients typically report lasting relief after just a few treatments.

Meditation and Spiritual Practice

Meditation can create a relaxation response in the body that promotes wellness. Spirituality is also an essential element of good health. Chronically ill individuals often feel somehow to blame for their illness, and sometimes feel that they are being punished or forgotten by GOD. Encourage clients to develop their spiritual and meditative resources. Meditation can be thinking about something pleasant and focusing on it. This could lead to increased relaxation and reduced tension. Many clients have received relief from chronic pain by focusing on the parts of the body that do not hurt. This serves two purposes, the first is to take attention away from the pain, the second is to allow the client to understand that only certain parts of the body are ill; the remainder is in pretty good shape. This could be akin to focusing on the donut, not the hole. Meditation can be anything from a trained mantra-utilization technique such as Transcendental Meditation, to repeating a phrase or praying the rosary. Most people respond to whatever meditation they are comfortable with and utilize regularly.

Spiritual practice is also important to those clients who are so inclined. Increasing spiritual or inspirational positive readings can be helpful in reducing stress and encouraging the body to heal. Insightful spiritual writers often discuss the issue of when bad things happen to us. By gaining insight into this normal part of living—bad things happen randomly—many individuals have improved their lives and health. There has also been extensive research on the power of distance prayer. In one study, groups of children who had leukemia were prayed for half way across the country and the control group in the study wasn't prayed for. Remarkably, the groups that both knew they were being prayed for or didn't know had significantly higher remission rates than the group that wasn't prayed for at all.

Genetic, stress, chemical, and physical assaults on the body are best healed in positive environments whether that be spiritual, meditational or anything else that brings comfort.

Positive Behavior

I cannot overemphasize the importance of positive health behaviors in the wellness and improved health of individuals suffering from chronic illness or pain. This does not mean a strict adherence to an inflexible regimen. One donut will probably not kill you. However, if you think about a behavior or food that you can choose to eat, such as apples or donuts, and 30 years of that food or behavior, you have a choice. Which road is more beneficial; one filled with donuts or one filled with apples? Where will a thirty-year road of donuts lead you? On the other hand, the occasional day without exercise or eating a fatty food will probably add to your enjoyment of life, and not detract from your health. Finding joy in life is a healing path for many individuals with chronic illness or pain. Reducing stress and increasing healthful habits are two resources in that goal.

Cutting Edge New Treatment

The drug Rituximab, which was previously used for cancer treatments, may treat rheumatoid arthritis in novel ways by more selectively targeting the B cells, which make antibodies that contribute to the disease process, according to research presented at the American College of Rheumatology Annual Scientific Meeting in New Orleans, Louisiana.

Multiple Sclerosis:

New Treatment

The National Institute of Allergy and Infectious Diseases (NIAID) reports a new treatment therapy for MS. This therapy is antigen-specific immunotherapy, which is based on a discovery by Dr. Lenardo and his colleagues that T-cells exposed to small amounts of the proteins making up the myelin sheaths are stimulated to attack the sheaths. T-cells exposed to large amounts of the same proteins will undergo a pre-programmed "self-destruct" sequence. (In fact, T-cells exposed to large amounts of any antigen -- a substance that provokes them to attack -- will self-destruct.) Therefore, introducing large amounts of myelin proteins into the body should remove the problematic T-cells and halt the disease, Dr. Lenardo explains. Furthermore, stem cells are showing promising results in the use of new treatments for MS. A study conducted at the San Raffaele Scientific Institute in Milan, Italy, showed that brain stem cells injected into the brains or veins of mice, repaired nerve damage similar to that seen in multiple sclerosis, according to Italian researchers who say their work could one day offer hope for treating the disease in humans.

Chapter 8

Stop the Madness:

Exercise and Diet

A proper diet and exercise can bring most individuals toward better health and improvement in chronic illness. American dietary habits are creating more illnesses and causing more obesity than ever before. The statistics of obesity in the United States are staggering compared to many other first world countries. It is estimated from the 1999-2000 National Health and Nutrition Examination Survey (NHANES) that an estimated 64 percent of U.S. adults are either overweight or obese.

Our culture has also become less active. Many individuals now find entertainment through the internet and television, which causes a chronically sedentary lifestyle leading to chronic health problems and increased obesity.

Our culture is also fast food, and fast-fix oriented. Nowhere else can you get a Big Gulp at 7-11 along with a Big Mac and super-sized fries at McDonald's and then drive through your local pharmacy to pick up your prescription of Lipitor. In that entire equation no one has to get out of the car. All of this overeating and under exercising is continuing to lead us down a path of chronic illness that may not be reversed unless our lifestyles and diet are changed forever. And in addition many of these dietary choices lead to even the most benign of problems like chronic heartburn. The highest number of prescriptions written in the United States is for Prilosec, a proton pump inhibitor used to fight acid reflux disease and heartburn, and the second-most prescribed drug on the market is Prozac, which is used primarily to treat depression.

    The American diet is filled with hydrogenated oil like margarine, hormones like those used in chickens and cattle to promote growth, refined sugars as in the case of candy and sodas, pesticides and preservatives, and fast food. Most of these foods would kill any lab rat within a week if they ate as much as Americans do and then just sat and looked at their exercise wheel. All of this is causing an epidemic number of people with high cholesterol, high-blood pressure, bowel difficulties, and malnutrition problems leading to illnesses like osteoporosis. The toxicity of many of these foods are creating or exacerbating already detrimental illnesses like autoimmune disease and stress-related illness.

    In addition to the lack of nutritional consciousness, many people smoke, drink many cups of coffee a day, and consume alcohol--which exacerbates illnesses that already plague our society. There are also possible toxins found in our meat supply alone. How many times have Americans turned on the television and heard another report of a child or elderly person dieing from

Understanding Autoimmune Disease and Stress-Related Illness

E-coli poisoning from contaminated hamburgers or some other form of beef. E-coli along with h-pylori have long been theorized to also contribute to the development of rheumatoid arthritis. The threat of mad cow disease is on the horizon for Americans, as many cows in England and now isolated cases in America have been found to have the disease. The threat of it spreading to America in epidemic proportions is eminent. Most modern day illnesses were borne out of animals and then later transmitted via fecal contamination or through consumption. For example, influenza was born out of cattle as well, and now we have SARS (Severe Acute Respiratory Syndrome) an illness causing acute respiratory illness leading to death. The culprit is held within animals, possibly chickens and rodents that carry the disease in China. Our meat supply inevitably carries many antibiotics and hormones in an effort to keep the cattle healthy and productive. Many chicken farmers use hormones in an effort to keep the chickens reproducing at high levels, which brings more profit to the chicken farmers. However, this could spell disaster for humans as we are being increasingly affected by these hormones and especially antibiotics, which are causing antibiotic resistance to such illnesses as salmonella.

Even when shopping and seeing signs for whole foods or organic foods, I am not sure what will kill me first—the pesticides on the whole foods or the lack of pesticides on the organic foods and the animal feces otherwise known as manure used to fertilize the organic foods.

These factors and the lack of exercise ultimately lead to poor health because our immune systems are unable to keep up with the task of eliminating all these toxins.

These poor habits, also lead to depression, anxiety and fatigue, which can ultimately lead to more chronic illness. This becomes a cycle of destruction. And the only way to stop this, is to change our diets and lifestyle.

By eliminating refined sugars, hydrogenated oils, meats with hormones or meats all together, pesticides, preservatives and avoiding fast food restaurants after work will start the path to better health. A study released by the University of Rijeka in Croatia, Department of Neurology, reports that after a study of MS patients and their diets, they found that most had a long history of consuming unpasteurized milk, animal fats, smoked meat and potatoes, which researchers believe are all risk factors, and could have an influence on the severity of primary demyelinization in a high-risk area for MS.

Another study out of the Department of Neurology at the Health Sciences University in Portland, Oregon, reported that saturated animal fats are directly involved in the development of MS. So it is imperative that MS patients avoid anything with saturated fats. It is thought by researchers that a vegetarian diet is beneficial for anyone affected by autoimmune disease and stress-related illness, because meat and animal fats have also been proven by research to exacerbate RA and Lupus symptoms as well.

All of these issues can be approached as poor dietary habits we have developed over time, so in their place we must put healthy habits at the forefront of our routine. Many researchers and scientists have done extensive research on the benefits of adding omega-3 and omega-6 essential fatty acids (EFA's). These are beneficial oils that are helpful for a variety of illnesses like heart disease, autoimmune illness, stress-related illness, depression and anxiety.

Fish oils and Evening Primrose oils help with fatigue and joint mobility. For those suffering illnesses like RA or Lupus and FMS, who have achy muscles and joints, these oils can act like a lubricant and they have anti-inflammatory properties that regulate prostaglandin hormones, which regulate inflammatory responses in the body.

For patients experiencing joint inflammation, EFA's are essential to help control the inflammatory process in the body. And for patients also experiencing chronic fatigue syndrome, EFA's are beneficial to counter fatigue.

A Mediterranean diet high in EFA's and olive oil has been thought to be beneficial for anyone experiencing autoimmune disease and stress-related illness. This type of diet not only reduces inflammatory reactions, it also provides relief from fatigue and associated illnesses that come with autoimmune disease like cognitive dysfunctions, as well as heart problems and internal organ failure, gastrointestinal problems like ulcerations caused from taking anti-inflammatory medications. Olive oil specifically has been proven to contribute to a better control of the hypertriglyceridemia accompanying diabetes and may reduce the risk of breast cancer and colorectum.

Research conducted by the University of Wisconsin-Madison—Department of Biochemistry suggests that in recent years there has been an effort to understand possible noncalcemic roles of vitamin D, including its role in the immune system and in particular, on T-cell mediated immunity. The significant role of vitamin D compounds as selective immunosuppressants is illustrated by their ability to either prevent or markedly suppress animal models of autoimmune disease. Vitamin D can either prevent or suppress experimental autoimmune encephalomyelitits, RA, lupus, type I diabetes, and inflammatory bowel disease. Studies suggest that vitamin D used daily at 400 I.U. will reduce the chance of developing MS by 46 percent. In a further research study it was revealed that sixteen percent of 25 people with multiple sclerosis (MS) given an average of 14,000 international units (IU) of vitamin D a day for a year suffered no relapses, according to Jodie Burton, MD, a neurologist at the University of Toronto. In contrast, close to 40% of 24 MS patients who took an average of 1,000 IU a day -- the amount

Understanding Autoimmune Disease and Stress-Related Illness

recommended by many MS specialists -- relapsed, she reported. Vitamin D appears to suppress the autoimmune responses thought to cause MS, Burton said. In MS, haywire T lymphocytes -- the cellular "generals" of the immune system -- order attacks on the myelin sheaths that surround and protect the brain cells. In people given high-dose vitamin D in the study, T cell activity dropped significantly. That didn't happen in people who took lower doses. Also, people taking high-dose vitamin D suffered 41% fewer relapses than the year before the study began, compared with 17% of those taking typical doses.

Researchers now have a better understanding of what role vitamin D plays in the development of MS. For people without a certain version of the gene Chromosome 6, the gene that plays a role in the development of multiple sclerosis, the risk for developing the disease is 1 in 1000. If someone has a certain variation of that gene, the risk increases to around 1 in 300 and 1 in 100 if a person has two copies of the gene variant. Now, researchers understand that during fetal development and very early childhood, certain proteins that are activated by vitamin D directly interact with the gene. Lack of vitamin D causes the gene to act in a way that increases the chances of developing multiple sclerosis.

In regards to patients experiencing RA who are taking methotrexate, it is postulated that they would benefit greatly from taking folate supplements. Several adverse affects are due to folate deficiencies, largely due to the antifolate properties of methotrexate. In order to reduce the adverse effects of methotrexate without compromising drug efficacy, folic acid supplementation is recommended. And folate, usually used in conjunction with B vitamins can also help in reducing the stress response. Patients who have chronic fatigue syndrome and fibromyalgia can benefit by the use of an overall B-complex that includes all the B vitamins as well as some ginseng for added energy and stress reduction. Ginseng also helps to rebuild exhausted adrenals caused from these illnesses or their medications. Licorice root has been proven effective in helping to fight adrenal burnout and also aids in digestive disorders that may accompany many harsh drugs used to treat autoimmune disease and stress-related illness.

    An overall balanced diet is also important. Adding selenium, zinc, vitamin C and a host of amino acids to the diet builds a strong immune system that is less apt to go awry. The building blocks of a healthy immune system are good nutrition. Nutrients will mobilize the immune system and stabilize it. A good multivitamin that has adequate amounts of the antioxidants A, E and C, and many other vitamins and minerals essential for good health will help with a balanced diet. If choosing a vegetarian diet, make sure to get adequate amounts of iron and B vitamins essential for energy. Other additional nutrients proven to help provide immune support include the Asian Shiitake mushrooms, and black or green tea. These provide strong antioxidant properties and powerful sustained immune support.

Other supplements that may bring some symptom relief with joint aches and pains, whether caused by RA, osteoarthritis or injury, include glucosamine and chondroitin. Patients injured due to a fall or just overexertion have benefited from these supplements.

In addition to a healthy diet, lifestyle changes such as adding exercise to your daily regiment may prove beneficial as well. Patients, who are dealing with the pain and inflammation of joints caused by RA or lupus, can benefit by doing water exercises. Water is a natural pain killer for these individuals because especially warm or hot water raises body temperature, which causes blood vessels to dilate and the individual will experience an increase in their circulation. Furthermore, it is a great buoyant exercise that won't overstress the joints and muscles and the water, whether cold or warm, is a great relaxant for anyone experiencing pain.

Water exercises, especially those usually offered by local community pools are a great way for RA, lupus and MS patients to increase stamina and build more muscle strength.

For those experiencing fibromyalgia and chronic fatigue, water exercises are also beneficial. And in addition to water exercises, aerobic fitness has benefited individuals who are experiencing CFS, by helping to increase stamina. For individuals who are experiencing on-going fibromyalgia symptoms or chronic fatigue, very light yoga and mediation has been useful at reducing stress and stiff muscles.

Experts caution patients with FMS, RA, lupus and MS about heavy weight lifting regiments as they can cause symptoms of these illnesses to flare up. Use light weights and caution.

For all of these recommendations, consult your personal physician or dietician before making any dietary or exercise changes. It is helpful to have a dietician formulate a specific diet for your condition and work with a physical therapist or personal trainer to design a specific and safe workout that will achieve maximum benefit.

Chapter 9

Preferred psychotherapies for working with autoimmune disease and stress-related illness

As with many illnesses, whether psychiatric or physiological, it is often difficult to determine which came first. As discussed in previous chapters, the stress response, and childhood abuse and neglect can lead to mental and physical illness. The question remains for researchers how much mental illness contributes, exacerbates or even causes some autoimmune diseases and stress-related illnesses. Research suggests that those who develop RA have a higher than average frequency of anxiety. Researchers, however, look at the history of many of the individuals who have developed fibromyalgia or RA, and realize that many of them were experiencing mental illness prior to the diagnosis. As with MS, many other autoimmune illnesses can take doctors many years to make a concrete diagnosis. Therefore, it is hard to determine if the chronic stress could have triggered the autoimmune reaction or if it were the result of the disease.

These questions are yet to be conclusively answered by researchers, but stress, which can include anxiety and depression, can make any illness seem unbearable and can further derail the immune system. This may or may not lead to an exacerbation of symptoms in autoimmune disease and stress-related patients.

Preferred Psychotherapies for Working with Autoimmune Disease

Because of possible ramifications of mental illness and chronic stress on the body's ability to fight disease, it is important to discuss intervention strategies that may be helpful for the patient to have more control over their disease and their accompanying symptoms. There are many approaches to helping the patient take control of their overall health.

Unlike working with individuals on anxiety and phobia issues, chronic illness doesn't go away. However, these are two different areas of study yet linked in many ways when dealing with fear and how to better cope with fear and anxiety of a newly diagnosed illness.

For example, a family that has just been told their child has MS, will typically go through many stages of dealing with that new crisis. Some of the stages may include anger, denial, bargaining, and then acceptance much like the stages of dealing with the imposing death of someone with a terminal illness. It is important to note that when a family or individual are given the news of an illness, many areas of development will be affected. It is important for their therapist to note many areas and new accommodations of one's life will need to be adjusted.

A member of a family who falls ill with a disease will put a new financial burden on the family. The individual may be in a wheelchair as a result of the new illness, and the family will need to make everything in the home and car handicap accessible, which adds more stress and financial burden upon the family.

The family may need to divide up different tasks in dealing with the patient and may be split between the parents and/or siblings.

The best type of therapeutic approach to use is one that is very cost effective, fast, easily applied and easily understood, and one that can better help the family and individual to cope with the crisis in a healthy, productive way. Because this situation is complex and often times very layered and complicated, it is important to deal with the situation head on. It is of no importance to spend time in a therapeutic setting delving into the family's past, because their lives will now be changed. It is also not cost-effective to delve into the past or the unconscious mind because it will serve no purpose to the here and now.

In examining effective therapeutic approaches, a cognitive-behavioral approach may be effective for an individual or family whose needs deal more directly with issues of anxiety and panic disorders around the new illness. The family may benefit from this therapeutic approach in many different ways by re-defining the role of the illness in their life as a challenge rather than an obstacle, which will help influence the family's behavior around the new illness. The behavior may be finding new activities for the individual to show mastery and help with self-esteem and confidence building. This may be important in keeping a positive outlook and approach to life with an illness.

Structural family therapy may be useful when dealing with poor communication and boundary setting. In structural

Preferred Psychotherapies for Working with Autoimmune Disease

family therapy more emphasis is placed on how the family is structured and how that affects other members of the family. With a sick child, the most useful part of this therapeutic approach might be to establish clear boundaries, so there is positive, effective communication between family members. It's also important for a parent not to triangulate with the sick child; the other spouse would feel left out or ganged up on. With an ill child, it would be important for the family to pay attention to everyone having equal time and input into solving issues that may arise.

Strategic and systemic family therapies could prove beneficial for a number of reasons. First, in using strategic family therapy, it is a short-term process of about 10 sessions, which makes it more affordable and possibly less physically and emotionally draining on both the sick individual and the family. In using this type of approach, it may be beneficial for the therapist to use reframing, to alter the perception of the negative consequences of an illness that has become a part of the family. In this situation give directives to the family. Telling the family to go slow and be patient with the process of coping with an extraordinary new situation (i.e. the illness) would help the family feel more at ease and less pressured to have instant change. Using different directives may help the family to feel less anxious and more relaxed through the process. It is also important to help the family to feel less frightened and more in control of their circumstances. It may be helpful in giving the family extra resources to work with outside of therapy. Letting them know of additional community support groups or organizations like Hospice would be helpful.

Enacting a certain situation that may arise as a result of having an ill family member may be helpful. The accustomed rules take over, and transactional components manifest themselves with intensity similar to that manifested in these transactions outside of the therapy session. This can be very helpful in letting the therapist become somewhat of a fly on the wall to observe how the family dynamics unravel.

Systemic family therapy treatment techniques of an ill child can also be beneficial. Bringing a positive connotation to a difficult and negative situation, may help the family change its perspective by re-framing the difficulties that can follow with the illness.

Strategic and systemic family therapies are especially helpful to families that have an ill child or other family member, because the process is very short and focused. It is easily comprehended and able to be applied to future issues, which will help the family to cope better as things arise.

There is the modality of solution-focused and narrative family therapies. For a family having difficulties dealing with their child falling ill, this type of therapy has superior techniques and concepts that can be presented in both these types of therapies.

Solution-focused and narrative family therapy is of particular importance and interest in dealing with ill family members, because it is about finding appropriate solutions instead of dealing and dwelling on the problem. Especially in the case of a medical crisis, the patient can become very overwhelmed with many opinions of their conditions and how to react to them. Sometimes it is helpful to externalize the problem or problems psychologically that surround such a crisis. The techniques in solution-focused therapy are helpful because this therapy lends itself to skeleton keys.

For example, the therapist may say, between now and next time we meet, observe what happens in your family that you want to discontinue. And the suggestion of doing something different encourages individuals and the family to explore the range of possibilities they have, rather than continue to do what they believe is correct. For instance, there is the example that a woman is complaining that her husband, a police detective, is staying out late every night with his friends. The message she received might be that her husband might want more mysterious behavior from her. Therefore, one night she hired a babysitter, rented a motel room, and stayed out until 5 a.m. Her husband came in at 2 a.m. nothing was said, but her husband began staying home at night.

Understanding Autoimmune Disease and Stress-Related Illness

That example is a great, non-aggressive way to confront a behavior to show the person in an indirect manner how their loved one is feeling or being treated. This can also be applied in the case of a sick child when no one decides to share chores in helping with the child or additional work that may need to be done. It may then be suggested that the person carrying most of the burden for unaccomplished work may just want to leave the chores and go to a movie and treat him or herself, while everyone else in the family has to deal with the natural consequences of not balancing the workload.

The technique of telling the family to pay attention to what they do when they overcome the temptation or urge to perform the symptom or some behavior associated with the complaint helps the family to realize an effective technique that can again be repeated with success. This guidance may help the family to understand and realize that they are in control of their issues.

Assigning homework to a family to realize different options or what others may do in a similar situation can help them to understand there are other avenues other than what have always been thought of or used in a similar situation. And the technique of all the family members or even just the ill family member writing down their frustrations and thoughts and then burning them can be very useful in helping with anger management and it also helps the individuals learn more about themselves.

A solution-focused approach is helpful in this case because it stresses that the family can change, and finds incidents where the family acts differently than usual, asking optimistic questions, and reinforcing small but specific movement. It also helps the family to look at the exceptions in behavior, which produces changes in families by challenging their worldview.

Overall, my selected choice between all these therapies in working with populations who are ill or family systems who have a child or spouse that is ill, would include a combination of cognitive-behavioral therapy where the family and patient can re-define the role of the illness in their life as a challenge rather than an obstacle. And solution focused and narrative family therapy, which focuses on skeleton keys, giving homework, and focusing on exceptions and giving compliments to boost self-esteem.

Other more hands-on therapies that have emerged recently would also include Eye Movement Desensitization-Reprocessing (EMDR), hypnosis, neural reprogramming, Thought Field Therapy (TFT), Emotion-Focused Therapy (EFT), biofeedback, and others, can be very powerful in healing the psychological issues of chronic illness and pain. However, the techniques themselves are not a single solution to a systemic problem. While all power techniques serve an important function in the overall treatment plan, incorporation of psycho-educational factors are equally necessary.

Education is a vital component in helping clients face their diagnosis. Educating the client to reduce stress, follow treatment regimens, increase positive thinking and lifestyle choices is essential to increase healing. Assisting in prioritizing the use of additional treatment resources such as massage, acupuncture, exercise, herbal therapies, meditation, spiritual activities, and improvement in relationship skills is also productive.

The client would be best served by a clinician who is kind, supportive, and well informed, as well as comfortable in challenging the client to reframe his or her response to the issues in life that may accompany the illness or pain. Clinicians should be non-judgmental regarding the issues the client is facing, as well as sensitive to the client's perceptions that others in his or her life may be judgmental. Regular examination of the issue is necessary to treat the underlying experience of the client. This is obvious in cases where the client may blame him or herself for the illness or pain. Clinicians may also want to focus on self-blame and reframing issues that encourage the client to understand that one can only do as much as can be done in a certain situation, and we never wish failure upon ourselves.

There can be secondary gain in the person's illness status. A lonely or otherwise distressed client may get attention or assistance in life when ill or in pain. Regardless of the clinician's treatment orientation, this issue should be dealt with in a positive, sympathetic manner. Happy, well-adjusted individuals do not wish to be ill. Individuals with secondary gain agendas are usually not ones with large resource pools from which they can seek assistance in handling disease. The clinician will have to treat this issue from the outset to enable improvement in the client's status.

Many individuals who have suffered a long-term chronic illness or been given a negative prognosis find the process of psychological healing to be frustratingly slow. This can be true even when successful power techniques are employed. The successful clinician will give attention to this issue. Encouraging the client to see progress in baby steps rather than huge leaps will also assist the client to establish a reality-based attitude. Timely checks on progress are also a means of reviewing the treatment plan and making desired adjustments.

Overall, in successful treatments, clients reduce stress, establish personally effective health regimens, adjust emotionally to the various effects of the illness, and find personally meaningful human and spiritual relationships. This process allows the client to reclaim his or her life. This does not necessarily mean that the presenting physical illness is cured. An individual who has lost an arm will not be getting his or her arm back. However, if the individual experiences chronic pain, depression, and anxiety regarding the loss of the limb, positive treatment will provide the client with successful adjustment and response to the tragedy and allow a positive self-image to emerge. Hopefully, clients will gain sufficient experience in responding to the illness or pain to gain insight and resources to respond to future challenges.

Clients can also have a tendency to overdo it when they start to feel some improvement. A common example would be an individual with chronic fatigue who experiences a remission of symptoms. It would not be unusual for the clinician to observe the individual take up a previous or new strenuous exercise regimen. Once again, the clinician should emphasize the importance of baby steps. The client could be encouraged to take baby steps in returning to both extensive exercise and heavy schedules. Otherwise, the strain on the body might produce a relapse. Alternatives to heavy exercise or work schedules should be explored early in the treatment plan. Yoga, stretching, Palates, bicycling, and swimming are often very effective in promoting physical fitness without placing undue strain on the body. Gradual increase in exercise time and difficulty is preferable to sudden changes. The philosophy of "no pain no gain" doesn't serve the health challenged individual. Satisfaction in regaining control of one's physical capacity can only be achieved by not harming the body during the process.

Preferred Psychotherapies for Working with Autoimmune Disease

Personal support systems and abrupt change will need close attention. In interpersonal relationships, the source of stress may be a family situation. Clients often have very strong feelings about family members and the personal systems in which they live. It is not unusual for a client to go home and simply stop doing an essential family function without allowing family members to adjust. By no longer fixing dinner, doing laundry, or going to work, and not allowing the family time to prepare for this change, the client is creating a stress-perpetuating crisis. Including family considerations and executive functioning in the treatment plan is essential. The clinician can educate the client in the necessity for an implementation plan for changes in family life.

Another situation that predicts failure in the wellness process is the sudden and cataclysmic change in long-term behaviors. This issue is evident in "new strategies" the client will take, such as becoming a vegetarian after years of poor diet choices. Many a refrigerator full of rotted organic and health promoting food has been thrown out due to the client's sudden decisions and lack of long term follow through. Again, gradual change with planned implementations predicts success in most cases. Self-discipline programs work best when gradual changes are introduced as part of the treatment plan.

Spiritual practices and beliefs have also proven helpful for those who are willing. For many years mental health workers have been somewhat shy in addressing the spiritual issues involved in wellness and psychological change. What is apparent in treating chronically ill individuals is that they may feel "dropped by GOD" or in some other way deserving of their affliction. Some religious belief systems include good health as a sign of a higher power's approval or blessing. It is cold comfort to add to this belief that GOD only gives us what we can handle. Rather than feed this self-defeating belief system, the clinician is encouraged to explore the client's spiritual belief system without evangelical agendas.

Clinicians are encouraged to explore the religious and spiritual resources available in the client's environment and establish contacts with leaders in the faith community who can communicate this positive message. These resources will provide an additional team member in the healing network available to the client and his or her family. The goal here is to assist the client in the restoration of trust and good will in his or her life. The client may need permission to be happy and healthy. He or she may feel that the permission needs to come from outside in the form of a religious blessing in addition to internal recognition. The resolution of spiritual issues can bring about an enormous surge in positive mental health.

Preferred Psychotherapies for Working with Autoimmune Disease

Perhaps the most important step in responding to the mental health challenges of chronic illness and pain is the use of new tools in life to prevent future stressors from overwhelming the client after the termination of treatment. This is not an issue of recidivism, but one of healing. The client will need to recognize that utilizing newly acquired skills to respond to this health crisis is not a time-limited experience. New wellness skills must be a regular part of future illness-prevention behaviors. In addition, some pain or illness may not be curable, however, if reoccurrence is experienced after remission, future self-blame will not serve the client any better than it has in the past. Indeed, there are some situations that cannot be resolved. This does not mean that needing assistance reflects failure. Asking for help when it is needed is a sign of good mental health.

Finally, clients and clinicians alike have their own unique responses to personal tragedies. The client brings his or her own personal beliefs, strengths and resources to the situation, just as the clinician. Traditional boundary making and keeping behaviors on the clinician's part may be challenged by clinical situations. In some cases, the clinician may find him or herself visiting clients in the hospital or at home. While these visits may be time consuming, and would in many situations be "billable" hours, I encourage clinicians to draw upon their resources of compassion and generosity when showing human kindness toward clients in crisis. Some of my best interventions have been birthday cards, chatty phone calls, home visits, and small gifts at important victories in the client's healing. These are parts of the natural interpersonal experience of one human being interacting with another. I cannot but reflect on my reaction in a training workshop where a licensed therapist asked the presenter if one should bill the client for attending the client's funeral. I was appalled. I am glad that I have been at the bedside of dying clients; often speaking to the unconscious client in his or her last days of life, or that I have gotten to know the client's family in the course of treatment. Sometimes, when dealing with autoimmune disease and chronic illness, the clinician must become part of the client's healing environment, not an outside observer. If the clinician has good personal boundaries upon which to draw, and the situation calls for this type of "personal touch" of compassion, I can find no clinical rationale for withholding signs of affection or human kindness.

Mental Health Treatment Modalities

EMDR, TFT, EFT, biofeedback, hypnosis, and other techniques have been used with great success in treating body-centered mental illness problems. The treatment of Post Traumatic Stress Disorder (PTSD) with EMDR has been well and thoroughly documented. EMDR is very effective in traumas because it is based on a seven phase integrative approach to help the client reprocess traumatic events into a less traumatic memory. EMDR can be very useful for several reasons. It is generally faster than traditional psychotherapies, it is easy to administer (with the use of client-produced tapping, or eye movement reprocessing administered by the clinician where the clients eyes follow the clinician finger while going through phases of the therapy), and it is highly effective and long lasting. It is the most researched and documented of the power therapy techniques. It is no longer considered an experimental technique due to its worldwide acceptance as a treatment of choice for many issues. For this reason, it is highly recommend for individuals experiencing autoimmune diseases, chronic pain, or stress-related illnesses and trauma. It is important to consult a trained, licensed therapist who is certified in EMDR and has extensive experience in treating body-centered illness.

How EMDR works to heal the body and brain

While the following description neither scientifically precise nor supported by specific neurophysiological research, has shown some rather stunning SPECT results with the use of EMDR in treating depression and anxiety. Evidently, EMDR produces physiological changes in the limbic area of the brain. It is thought that it restores the amygdala and hippocampus areas of the brain to more normal functioning. This can be seen in changes in the sizes of these two centers of stress or information processing.

Chronically stressed limbic systems have smaller amygdala and hippocampus areas than non-stressed brains.

The use of hypnosis and biofeedback are also some of the most utilized power techniques. Indeed, many therapists use them extensively, by referral, prior to learning EMDR. They each have their own uses, especially in areas of relaxation training, positive reinforcement of improved health behaviors (such as stopping smoking and reducing intake of drug or alcohol), and they can be very effective in reducing chronic pain. Relaxation training cannot be overemphasized. Many autoimmune diseases have been shown to respond to relaxation therapies. For example, in the treatment of MS, decreasing stressors can decrease the exacerbation of flare-ups and lesion formation. Because of this, it is essential therefore for the client and therapist to understand the psychosocial history of the client.

Sadly, there is some evidence that poorly conducted psychosocial histories and subsequent treatment can induce false memories in some clients. I strongly advise clients that the use of any of the above techniques is not done with a goal of determining if someone was abused or molested as a child or adult. All memories or thoughts experienced in treatment should be considered "dream-like" in nature and not be used as "proof" of past harms.

Chapter 10

Additional Resources

National Institute of Arthritis and Musculoskeletal and Skin Diseases Information Clearinghouse

NIAMS/National Institutes of Health

1 AMS Circle

Bethesda, MD 20892-3675

(301) 495-4484 or (877) 22-NIAMS (toll free)

TTY: (301) 565-2966

Fax: (301) 718-6366

World Wide Web address: http://www.niams.nih.gov/

The National Institute of Arthritis and Musculoskeletal and Skin Diseases Information Clearinghouse is a public service sponsored by the NIAMS that provides health information and information sources. The clearinghouse provides information on lupus. Fact sheets, additional information, and research updates can also be found on the NIAMS Web site at http://www.niams.nih.gov/.

Additional Resources

Association of Rheumatology Health Professionals, American College of Rheumatology

1800 Century Place, Suite 250

Atlanta, GA 30345

(404) 633-3777

Fax: (404) 633-1870

World Wide Web address: http://www.rheumatology.org/

The American College of Rheumatology (ACR) is an organization of doctors and associated health professionals who specialize in arthritis and related diseases of the bones, joints, and muscles. The Association of Rheumatology Health Professionals, a division of ACR, aims to enhance the knowledge and skills of rheumatology health professionals and to promote their involvement in rheumatology research, education, and quality patient care. The association also works to advance and promote basic and continuing education in rheumatology for health professionals who provide care to people with rheumatic diseases.

Additional Resources

Lupus Foundation of America (LFA), Inc.

1300 Piccard Drive, Suite 200

Rockville, MD 20850

(301) 670-9292

(800) 558-0121

or your local chapter, listed in the telephone directory

Web address: http://www.lupus.org/

This is the main voluntary organization devoted to lupus. The LFA assists local chapters in providing services to people with lupus, works to educate the public about lupus, and supports lupus research. Through a network of more than 500 branches and support groups, the chapters provide education through information and referral services, health fairs, newsletters, publications, and seminars. Chapters provide support to people with lupus, their families, and friends through support group meetings, hospital visits, and telephone help lines.

Additional Resources

SLE Foundation, Inc.

149 Madison Avenue, Suite 205

New York, NY 10016

(212) 685-4118

World Wide Web address: http://www.lupusny.org/

The foundation supports and encourages medical research to find the cause and cure of lupus and improve its diagnosis and treatment. It also provides a wide variety of services to help patients with lupus and their families. In addition, this voluntary organization conducts a broad-based public education program to raise awareness of lupus and increase understanding of this serious, chronic, autoimmune disease.

Arthritis Foundation

1330 West Peachtree Street

Atlanta, GA 30309

(404) 872-7100

Additional Resources

(800) 283-7800, or call your local chapter (listed in the telephone directory)

World Wide Web address: http://www.arthritis.org/

The Arthritis Foundation is the major voluntary organization devoted to supporting arthritis research and providing educational and other services to individuals with arthritis. It publishes free pamphlets and a magazine for members on all types of arthritis. It also provides up-to-date information on research and treatment, nutrition, alternative therapies, and self-management strategies. Chapters nationwide offer exercise programs, classes, support groups, physician referral services, and free literature. For more information, call your local chapter, listed in the white pages of the phone book, or contact the Arthritis Foundation at the above address.

Alliance for Lupus Research, Inc.

1270 Avenue of the Americas, Suite 609

New York, NY 10020

(212) 218-2840

The Alliance for Lupus Research, Inc. (ALR), is a nonprofit organization devoted exclusively to the support of promising research for the prevention, treatment, and cure of lupus. Through accelerated, focused, goal-oriented research programs, the ALR aims to promote basic and clinical sciences to achieve major advances leading to a better understanding of the cause of lupus.

National CFS Patient Organizations

Chronic Fatigue and Immune Dysfunction Syndrome Association of America

P.O. Box 220398

Charlotte, NC 28222

1-800-442-3437

http://www.cfids.org

National Chronic Fatigue Syndrome and Fibromyalgia Association

P.O. Box 18426

Kansas City, MO 64133

816-313-2000

Health Professional Organizations

American Association for Chronic Fatigue Syndrome

325 Ninth Avenue

Box 359780

Seattle, WA 98104

206-781-3544

Where Can People Get More Information About Fibromyalgia?

- Arthritis Foundation

    1330 West Peachtree Street

    Atlanta, GA 30309

    404/872-7100

Additional Resources

800/283-7800 or call your local chapter (listed in the telephone directory)

World Wide Web address: http://www.arthritis.org

This is the main voluntary organization devoted to all forms of arthritis. The Foundation publishes a pamphlet on fibrositis. Single copies are free with a self-addressed stamped envelope. The Foundation also can provide physician referrals.

- Fibromyalgia Network

    P.O. Box 31750

    Tucson, AZ 85751-1750

    800/853-2929

    Contact: Ms. Kristin Thorson

- Fibromyalgia Partnership (formerly Fibromyalgia Association of Greater Washington)

    140 Zinn Way

    Linden, VA 22642-5609

    (toll free) 866/725-4404

Additional Resources

Fax: 540-622-2998

World Wide Web address: http://www.fmpartnership.org

- National Fibromyalgia Awareness Campaign (NFAC)

    2415 N. River Trail Road, Suite 200

    Orange, CA 92865

    714/921-0150

    Fax: 714/921-8139

These are the main organizations devoted to fibromyalgia. They publish newsletters and provide pamphlets on the disease.

National Multiple Sclerosis Society

733 Third Avenue

6th Floor

New York, NY 10017-3288

nat@nmss.org

http://www.nationalmssociety.org

Tel: 212-986-3240 800-344-4867 Fax: 212-986-7981

Funds research, helps families stay together, provides accurate and up-to-date information, helps with employment issues, offers free counseling, runs self-help groups, advocates for people with disabilities, and provides referrals to medical professionals.

Multiple Sclerosis Association of America

706 Haddonfield Road

Cherry Hill, NJ 08002

msaa@msaa.com

http://www.msaa.com

Tel: 856-488-4500 800-532-7667

Fax: 856-661-9797

National, non-profit organization dedicated to enhancing the quality of life for those affected by multiple sclerosis. MSAA provides ongoing support and direct services to individuals with MS and their families and works to promote a greater understanding of the needs and challenges of those who face physical obstacles.

Additional Resources

Multiple Sclerosis Foundation

6350 North Andrews Avenue

Ft. Lauderdale, FL 33309-2130

support@msfocus.org

http://www.msfocus.org

Tel: 954-776-6805 888-MSFocus (673-6287)

Fax: 954-351-0630

Dedicated to helping people with MS, the Multiple Sclerosis Foundation offers a wide array of free services including: national toll-free support, educational programs, homecare, support groups, assistive technology, publications, a comprehensive website, and more programs to improve the quality of life for those affected by MS.

Other voluntary health agencies that can provide general information on MS or symptoms associated with MS include:

National Ataxia Foundation (NAF)

2600 Fernbrook Lane

Additional Resources

Suite 119

Minneapolis, MN 55447-4752

naf@ataxia.org

http://www.ataxia.org

Tel: 763-553-0020

Fax: 763-553-0167

Encourages and supports research into the hereditary ataxias, a group of chronic and progressive neurological disorders affecting coordination. Sponsors chapters and support groups throughout the U.S.A. and Canada. Publishes a quarterly newsletter and educational literature on the various forms of ataxia.

International Essential Tremor Foundation

P.O. Box 14005

Lenexa, KS 66285-4005

staff@essentialtremor.org

http://www.essentialtremor.org

Tel: 913-341-3880 888-387-3667

Additional Resources

Provides educational information, funds research in tremor disorders, and offers services and support to individuals diagnosed with essential tremor, their families, and health care providers. Information and support includes a quarterly newsletter, support groups, and physician information and referrals.

Well Spouse Foundation

63 West Main Street Suite H

732-577-8644

Freehold, NJ 07728

info@wellspouse.org

http://www.wellspouse.org

Tel: 800-838-0879 732-577-8899

Fax: 732-577-8644

International non-profit organization whose mission is to provide emotional support to, raise consciousness about, and advocate for the spouses/partners and children of the chronically ill and/or disabled.

Additional Resources

American Autoimmune Related Diseases Association

22100 Gratiot Avenue

Eastpointe

East Detroit, MI 48201-2227

aarda@aol.com

http://www.aarda.org

Tel: 586-776-3900 800-598-4668

Fax: 586-776-3903

National organization that works to alleviate suffering and the socioeconomic impact of autoimmunity. Dedicated to the eradication of autoimmune diseases through fostering and facilitating collaboration in the areas of education, research, and patient services.

Paralyzed Veterans of America (PVA)

801 18th Street, NW

Washington, DC 20006-3517

info@pva.org

Additional Resources

http://www.pva.org

Tel: 202-USA-1300 (872-1300) 800-424-8200

Fax: 202-785-4452

Works to help members and their families, as well as all veterans and people with disabilities. Offers expertise on a wide variety of issues involving the special needs of veterans of the armed forces who have experienced spinal cord dysfunction.

Boston Cure Project for MS

13 Belton Street

Arlington, MA 02474

info@bostoncure.org

http://www.bostoncure.org

Tel: 781-788-0880

Fax: 781-788-8188

Non-profit organization dedicated to the creation and execution of a national plan to cure MS.

Additional Resources

National Organization for Rare Disorders (NORD)

P.O. Box 1968

(55 Kenosia Avenue)

Danbury, CT 06813-1968

orphan@rarediseases.org

http://www.rarediseases.org

Tel: 203-744-0100 Voice Mail 800-999-NORD (6673)

Fax: 203-798-2291

Federation of voluntary health organizations dedicated to helping people with rare "orphan" diseases and assisting the organizations that serve them. Committed to the identification, treatment, and cure of rare disorders through programs of education, advocacy, research, and service.

In addition to the NINDS, there are several other Federal Government agencies that may be able to provide information on MS. They are the:

Additional Resources

Food and Drug Administration (FDA)

5600 Fishers Lane

CDER-HFD-210

Rockville, MD 20857

http://www.fda.gov

Tel: 301-827-4573 888-INFO-FDA (463-6332)

National Rehabilitation Information Center (NARIC)

4200 Forbes Boulevard

Suite 202

Lanham, MD 20706-4829

naricinfo@heitechservices.com

http://www.naric.com

Tel: 301-562-2400 800-346-2742

Fax: 301-562-2401

Multiple Sclerosis Research Centers:

To find better ways to prevent and treat multiple sclerosis, the NINDS research program supports a broad spectrum of studies

Additional Resources

by investigators at leading biomedical research institutions across the country. Information on research activities at these centers may be obtained by contacting the principal investigators listed below.

Robert Lazzarini, Ph.D.

Brookdale Center for Molecular Biology, Box 1126

Mount Sinai Medical Center

One Gustave L. Levi Place

New York, NY 10029

212-241-4272

Robert P. Lisak, M.D.

Department of Neurology

Wayne State University

4201 St. Antoine Street, 6E/UHC

Detroit, MI 48201

313-577-1249

Additional Resources

Stephen Miller, Ph.D.

Department of Microbiology-Immunology

Northwestern University Medical School

303 East Chicago Avenue

Chicago, IL 60611

312-503-7674

Cedric Raine, M.D.

Albert Einstein College of Medicine of

Yeshiva University

1300 Morris Park Avenue

Bronx, NY 10461

718-430-2495

*A. M. Rostami, M.D., Ph.D.

Department of Neurology

University of Pennsylvania Medical Center

3400 Spruce Street

Philadelphia, PA 19104

215-662-6557

Additional Resources

Stephen Stohlman, Ph.D.

Department of Neurology

University of Southern California

1333 San Pablo Street, Room MCH-142

Los Angeles, CA 90033

213-342-1058

John N. Whitaker, M.D.

Department of Neurology

University of Alabama at Birmingham

Birmingham, AL 35294-0007

205-934-2402

References:

Introduction and Chapter 1

- *American Autoimmune Related Diseases Association*
- *Institute of Arthritis and Musculoskeletal and Skin Disease*
- *National Institutes of Health*

References

Chapters 2

Barsky, A. J., & Borus, J. F. (1999). Functional Somatic Syndromes. *Annals of Internal Medicine, 130*, 910-921.

Demitrack, M. A., & Crofford, L. J. (1998). Evidence for and Pathophysiologic Implications of Hypothalamic-Pituitary-Adrenal Axis Dysregulation in Fibromyalgia and Chronic Fatigue Syndrome. *Annals of the New York Academy of Sciences, 840*, 684-697.

Deuschle, M., Weber, B., Colla, M., Depner, M., & Heuser, I. (1998). Effects of Major Depression, Aging and Gender Upon Calculated Diurnal Free Plasma Cortisol Concentrations: A Re-evaluation Study. *Stress, 2*, 281-287.

Kaplan, K. H., Goldenberg, D. L., & Galvin-Nadeau, M. (1993). The Impact of a Meditation-Based Stress Reduction Program on Fibromyalgia. *General Hospital Phychiatry, 15*, 284-289.

References

Lechin, F., Van Der Dijs, B., Lechin, A., Orozco, B., Lechin, M., Baez, S., Rada, I., Leon, G., & Acosta, E. (1994). Plasma Neurotransmitters and Cortisol in Chronic Illness: Role of Stress. *Journal of Medicine*, *25*, 181-192.

Marchetti, B., Morale, M. C., Testa, N., Tirolo, C., Caniglia, S., Amor, S., Dijkstra, C. D., & Barden, N. (2001). Stress, the Immune System and Vulnerability to Degenerative Disorders of the Central Nervous System in Transgenic Mice Expressing Glucocorticoid Receptor Antisense RNA. *Brain Research - Brain Research Reviews*, *37*, 259-272.

Mohr, D. C., Goodkin, D. E., Nelson, S., Cox, D., & Weiner, M. (2002). Moderating Effects of Coping on the Relationship Between Stress and the Developement of new Brain Lesions in Multiple Sclerosis. *Psychosomatic Medicine*, *64*, 803-809.

Schwartz, C. E., Foley, F. W., Rao, S. M., Bernardin, L. J., Lee, H., & Genderson, M. W. (1999). Stress and Course of

References

Disease in Multiple Sclerosis. *Behavioral Medicine*, *25*, 110-116.

Straub, R. H., Scholmerich, J., & Zietz, B. (2000). Replacement Therapy with DHEA plus Corticosteroids in Patients with Chronic Inflammatory Diseases--Substitutes of Adrenal and Sex Hormones. *Zeitschrift fur Rheumatologie*, *59*, 108-118.

Yang, Q. (2000). Central Control of the Hypothalamic-Pituitary-Adrenocortical Axis for Stress Reponse. *Sheng Li Ko Hsueh Chin Chan*, *31*, 222-226.

References

Chapter 3

- *Regis University*
- *Colorado State University*

References

Chapter 4

Berkowitz, L. (1984). Some Effects of Thought on Anti-and Pro-Social Influences of Media Events A Cog-Neoassociation Analysis. *Psychological Bulletin, 95*, 410-427.

Carlson, V., Cicchetti, D., Barnett, D., & Braunwald, K. (1989). Disorganized/Disoriented Attachment Relationships in Maltreated Infants. *Development Psychology, 25*, 525-531.

Charney, D. S., Deutch, A. Y., Krystal, J. H., Southwick, S. M., & Davis, M. (1993). Psychobiological Mechanisms of Post-Traumatic Stress Disorder. *Archives of General Psychiatry, 50*, 294-305.

Crawford, C. (1994). *No Safe Place-The Legacy of Family Violence*. New York: Station Hill Press.

Dorr, A., & Kovanic, P. (1981). *Some of the People Some of the Time-but Which People? Televised Violence and its Effects.* E. L. Palmer, & A. Dorr (Eds.). New York: Academic Press.

References

Finestone, H. M., Stenn, P., Davies, F., Stalker, C., Fry, R., & Koumanis, J. (2000). Chronic Pain and Health Care Utilization in Women with a History of Childhood Sexual Abuse. *Child Abuse & Neglect, 24*, 547-556.

Gunter, B. (1990). *Does Television Influence Aggressive Behaviour? Children and Television: The One Eyed Monster?*. London: Routledge.

Johnston, V. S., & Wang, X. T. (1991). The Relationship Between Menstrual Phase and the P3 Component of ERPs. *Psychophysiology, 38*, 400-409.

Josephson, W. L. (1987). Television Violence and Children's Aggression: Testing the Priming, Social Script and Disinhibition Predictions. *Journal of Personality and Social Psychology, 53*, 882-890.

Kestenbaum, R., & Nelson, C. A. (1992). Neural and Behavioral Correlates of Emotion Recognition in Children and Adults. *Journal of Experimental Child Psychology, 54*, 1-18.

References

Miller, G. A., Simon, R. F., & Lang, P. J. (1984). Electrocortical Measures in Information Processing Deficits in Anhedonia. *Annals of the New York Academy of Sciences, 425*, 598-602.

Parliamentary Office of Science and Technology . (1993) Screen Violence. Information for Members, Briefing Note 44 , London, P.O.S.T.

Pennell, A., & Browne, K. (1998). Film Violence and Young Offenders. *Aggression and Violent Behavior, 1*, 13-28.

Pollak, S. (1997). Conginitive Brain Event-Related Potentials and Emotion Processing in Maltreated Children. *Child Development, 5*, 773-787.

Rossman, B. B. R. (1998). Descartes's Error and Posttraumatic Stress Disorder: Cognition and Emotion in Children Who Are Exposed to Parental Violence. *The American Psychological Association, 11*, 223-251.

Santrock, J. W. (1999). *Life-Span Development* (7th ed.). United States of America: McGraw-Hill Companies, Inc.

References

Sappington, A. A. (2000). Childhood Abuse As a Possible Locus For Early Intervention Into Problems of Violence and Psychopathology. *Aggression and Violent Behavior, 3,* 255-266.

Thomas, M., Horton, R. W., Lippencott, E. C., & Drabman, R. S. (1997). Desensitisation to Portrayals of Real-Life Aggression as a Function of Exposure to Television Violence. *Journal of Personality and Social Psychology, 35,* 450-458.

Vander Kolk, B. A. (1994). The Body Keeps Score: Memory and the Evolving Psychobiology of Post-Traumatic Stress. *Harvard Review of Psychiatry, 1,* 253-265.

Van Houdenhove, B., Neerinckx, E., Lysens, R., Vertommen, H., Van Houdenhove, L., Onghena, P., Westhovens, R., D'Hooghe, M. B. (2001) Victimization in Chronic Fatigue Syndrome and Fibromyalgia in Tertiary Care: A Controlled Study on Prevalence and Characteristics. *Psychosomatics, 42,* 21-28.

References

Walker, E. A., Keegan, D., Gardner, G., Sullivan, M., Bernstein, D., & Katon, W. J. (1997). Psychosocial Factors in Fibromyalgia Compared with Rheumatoid Arthritis: II. Sexual, Physical, and Emotional Abuse and Neglect. *Psychosomatic Medicine, 59,* 572-577.

Williamson, S., Timothy, J. H., & Hare, R. D. (1991). Abnormal Processing of Affective Words by Psychopaths. *Psychophysiology, 28,* 260-273.

Winfield, J. B. (1999). Pain in Fibromyalgia. *Rheumatic Diseases Clinics of North America, 25,* 55-79.

References

Chapters 5-6

Al-Allaf, A. W., Dunbar, K. L., Hallum, N. S., Nosratzadek. B., Templeton. L.D. & Pullar, T. (2002). A case-control study examining the role of physical trauma in the onset of fibromyalgia syndrome. Rheumatology, 41(4), 450-453.

Amen, D. G. (2003). EMDR International Associates Conference, Denver, Colorado, September 19,

El-Miedany, Y. M., & El-Rasheed, A. H. (2002).

Common Disorder in Depression in Rheumatoid Arthritis *Joint, Bone, Spine: Revue of Rheumatism*, *69*, 300-306.

Fischler, B., Cluydts, R., De Gucht, Y., Kaufman, L., & DeMeirleir, K. (1997). Generalized Anxiety Disorder in Chronic Fatigue Syndrome. *Acta Psychiatrica Scandinavica*, *95*, 405-413.

References

Katon, W., Sullivan, M., & Walker, E. (2001). Medical Symptoms Without Identified Pathology: Relationship to Psychiatric Disorders, Childhood and Adult Trauma, and Personality Traits. *Annals of Internal Medicine, 134,* 917-925.

Walker, E. A., Keegan, D., Gardner, G., Sullivan, M., Katon, W. J., & Bernstein, D. (1997). Psychosocial Factors in Fibromyalgia Compared with Rheumatoid Arthritis: I. Psychiatric Diagnoses and Functional Disability. *Psychosomatic Medicine, 59,* 565-571.

References

Chapter 7

New Hope for Vaccine to Fight Rheumatoid Arthritis, Other Autoimmune Diseases. (2002). *Journal of Immunology*.

References

Chapter 8

Aerobic Fitness Effects in Fibromyalgia. (2003). *Journal of Rheumatology, 30,* 1060-1090.

Alarcan de la Lastra, C., Barranco, M. D., Motilva, V., & Herrerias, J.M. (2001). Mediterranean Diet and Health: Biological Importance of Olive Oil. *Curr Pharm Des, 7,* 933-950.

Beren, J., Diener-West, M., Hill, S. L., & Rose, N. R. (2001). Effect of Pre-Loading Oral Glucosamine HCI/Chondrotin Sulfate/Manganese Ascorbate Combination on Experimental Arthritis in Rats. *Exp Biol Med, 226,* 144-151.

Calder, P. C. (2001). Polyunsaturated Fatty Acids, Inflammation, and Immunity. *Lipids, 36,* 1007-1024.

Clark, W. F., Parbtani, A., Huff, M.W., Spanner, E., de Salis, H., Chin-Yee, I., Philbrick, D. J., Holub, B.J. (1995). Flaxseed: A Potential Treatment for Lupus Nephritis. *Kidney Int, 48,* 475-480.

References

Danao-Camara, T. C., & Shintani, T. T. (1999). The Dietary Treatment of Infammatory Arthritis: Case Reports and Review of the Literature. *Hawaii Med Journal, 58*, 126-131.

Deluca, H. F., & Cantorna, M.T. (2001). Vitamin D: Its Role and Uses in Immunology. *FASEB J, 15*, 2579-2585.

Endresen, G. K., & Husby, G. (2001). Folate Supplementation During Methotrexate Treatment of Patients with Rheumatoid Arthritis. An Update and Proposals for Guidelines. *Scand J Rheumatology, 30*, 129-134.

Grant, W. B. (2000). The Role of Meat in the Expression of Rheumatoid Arthritis. *Britian Journal of Nutrition, 84*, 589-595.

Grant, W. B. (2000). The Role of Meat in the Expression of Rheumatoid Arthritis. *British Journal of Nutrition, 84*, 589-595.

References

Hakkinen, S., Adlercreutz, H., & Laakso, J. (2000). Antioxidants in Vegan Diet and Rheumatic Disorders. *Toxicology, 115*, 45-53.

Minami, Y., Sasaki, T., Arai, Y., Kurisu Y., Hisamichi, S. (2003). Diet and Systemic Lupus Erythematosus: A 4 Year Prospective Study of Japanese Patients. *Journal of Rheumatology, 30*, 747-754.

McDougall, J., Bruce B., Spiller, G., Westerdahl, J., McDougall, M. (2002). Effects of a Very Low-Fat, Vegan Diet in Subjects with Rheumatoid Arthritis. *J Altern Complement Med, 8*, 71-75.

Racciatti, D., Guagnano, M.T., Vecchiet, J., De Remigis, P.L., Pizzigallo, E., Della Vecchia R., Di Sciascio, T., Merlitti, D., Sensi, S. (2001). Chronic Fatigue Syndrome: Circadian Rhythm and Hypothalamus-Pituitary-Adrenal (HPA) Axis Impairment. *Int Jounal of Pharamocolgy, 14*, 11-15.

References

Sepcic, J., Mesaros, E., Materljan, E., Sepic-Grahovac, D.(1993). Nutritional Factors and Multiple Sclerosis in Gorski Kotar, Croatia. *Neuroepidemiology, 12*, 234-240.

Swank, R. L. (1991). Multiple Sclerosis: Fat-Oil Relationship. *Nutrition, 7*, 368-376.

Valim V., Oliveira, L., Suda, A., Silva, L., Assis, M.D., Neto, T.B., Feldman, D., & Natour, J. (2003). Aerobic Fitness Effects in Fibromyalgia. *Journal of Rheumatology, 30*, 1060-1090.

Venkatraman, J. T., & Chu, W.C. (1999). Effects of Dietary Omega-3 and Omega-6 Lipids and Vitamin E on Serum Cytokines, Lipid Mediators and anti-DNA Antibodies in a Mouse Model for Rheumatoid Arthritis. *J Am Coll Nutu, 18*, 602-613.

References

Chapter 9

Fishman, H., & Minuchin, S. (1981). *Family Therapy Techniques*. Cambridge, MA: Harvard University Press.

Gladding, S. T. (1997). *Family Therapy: History, Theory and Practice* (2nd ed.). New Jersey: Prentice-Hall, Inc.

Mohr, D. C., Goodkin, D. E., Nelson, S., Cox, D., & Weiner, M. (2002). Moderating effects of coping on the relationship between stress and the development of new brain lesions in multiple sclerosis. *Psychosomatic Medicine, 64(5), 803-809.*

Shapiro, F. (1988). Eye movement desensitization: A new treatment for post-traumatic stress disorder. *Journal of Behavior Therapy and Experimental Psychiatry, 20, pp. 211-217.*